Medical Interviews Professional Development

An essential handbook for the junior doctor

Second Edition

Chinmoy K Maity MBBS, DTM&H & MD (Calcutta); MRCP (London)
Specialist Registrar in Geriatrics and General Internal Medicine
Royal Liverpool University Hospital

Foreword by

Jeremy R Playfer
Consultant Geriatrician
Royal Liverpool and Broadgreen University Hospitals
President, British Geriatrics Society

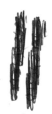

Radcliffe Publishing
Oxford • Seattle

Radcliffe Publishing Ltd
18 Marcham Road
Abingdon
Oxon OX14 1AA
United Kingdom

www.radcliffe-oxford.com
Electronic catalogue and worldwide online ordering facility.

© 2006 Chinmoy K Maity

Reprinted 2008

Chinmoy K Maity has asserted his right under the Copyright, Designs and Patents Act 1998 to be identified as author of this work.

First Edition 2004 (published by Sandpiper Publishing)

All rights reserved. No part of this publication may be reproduced, stored in a retrieval system or transmitted, in any form or by any means, electronic, mechanical, photo-copying, recording or otherwise without the prior permission of the copyright owner.

British Library Cataloguing in Publication Data

A catalogue record for this book is available from the British Library.

ISBN-10: 1 84619 080 0
ISBN-13: 978 1 84619 080 3

Typeset by Ann Buchan (Typesetters), Middlesex
Printed and bound by TJI Digital, Padstow, Cornwall

Contents

Foreword

I am delighted to provide the foreword to the second edition of Dr Maity's excellent handbook for junior doctors on *Medical Interviews and Professional Development*. The first edition of the book deservedly received excellent recommendations and reviews from leading lights in our profession. For once a really useful book, which is written very clearly and does not assume previous knowledge. It deals with those non-clinical areas of medicine, which are often not found in other textbooks, that are vital to effective clinical practice. The focus is very much on topics which tend to be concentrated on in interviews to select people for higher training or for consultant jobs. All of us often have embarrassing hiatuses or gaps in this knowledge. How often have any of us stopped to think of what a particular abbreviation stands for and had difficulty recalling its original meaning? This book leaps to our aid giving clear concise descriptions. All abbreviations are fully annotated and explained.

I am in the fortunate position that I am unlikely to face another interview committee! However, it is a very important part of my job to prepare the junior staff working with me to progress in their careers. An essential skill is negotiating the interview process.

I personally will be buying copies of this edition so that in addition to the limited advice I can give people, they can have a book that will adequately prepare them for the ordeal of interviews.

Medical publishing is changing greatly. We are so used to getting the information we need from the Internet, it is easy to neglect the value and purpose of guidebooks. I think the acquisition of this book will be extremely helpful to all junior doctors. Having a book to hand, which is so attractive, well thought out and written will add an edge to the individual's confidence. The new edition maps out important non-clinical areas of our professional life and helps us acquire knowledge of these in a systematic rather than the usual haphazard way.

Dr Maity is to be congratulated on an excellent piece of scholarship, which has arisen naturally out of his experiences as a trainee. The publication deserves every success and I suspect that those junior doctors who acquire it will regard it as one of the most valuable investments they have made. It will certainly aid them in their progress through the profession.

Dr Jeremy R Playfer MD, FRCP
Consultant Physician in Geriatric Medicine
Royal Liverpool University Hospital
President of the British Geriatrics Society
April 2006

About the author

Dr Chinmoy Kumar Maity MBBS, DTM&H, MD, MRCP (UK) graduated from the premier medical institute of Asia (Calcutta Medical College, India). After completing his postgraduate training in Tropical Medicine and General Internal Medicine in Calcutta, he came to the United Kingdom for further training in 1996. His initial training was done in Peterborough, South Wales and Hammersmith. He is now working as a type 1 Specialist Registrar in Geriatrics and General Internal Medicine at Royal Liverpool University Hospital.

Chinmoy is a natural born teacher and has been very keen on both literary and medical writing from an early age. His first book, the first edition of this book, has been extensively reviewed and well accepted across the United Kingdom.

Preface to the second edition

Writing the preface of a book is one of the most pleasurable experiences in an author's life, which could probably be compared only with that of a mother who has just given birth to a healthy baby after long gestation and a prolonged labour. Throughout the whole book I have tried to depict the journey of a junior doctor through a series of hurdles along the career pathway.

The first edition of this book has been extensively reviewed and well received across the United Kingdom. I have received numerous constructive criticisms and suggestions from my colleagues and friends, which form the basis of this second edition. All the chapters have been thoroughly revised and updated. A few new chapters entitled 'Medical ethics', 'Medico-social issues' and all chapters under the 'Medico-legal issues' section have been added to cover almost all aspects of medical interviews and professional development of not only junior doctors, but also nurses.

The chapters have been reoriented and for practical reasons they have been divided into five sections, although they are not watertight compartments. Useful appendices and a detailed index are also added features in this new edition. I hope the readers will find it useful.

Chinmoy K Maity
April 2006

Preface to the first edition

The main reason behind my attempt in writing this handbook is the painful experiences and difficulties I faced as a junior doctor at different levels of my career in getting information on the topics discussed here. The topics discussed in this book are very topical, quite useful in everyday practice and often questions are asked on these topics in interviews. There are a number of good books on each of these issues written by renowned authors in their respective fields. However, as a busy junior doctor or a clinician, we do not have the time to go through so much detail and practically we do not need them in great detail in our day-to-day practice. The main purpose of this handbook is to give a brief but overall view on these topics to deal with them confidently in everyday practice. Nevertheless, for more detailed information on any particular topic, the reader is referred to relevant references given at the end of the book. Finally, my humble attempt will be considered as a success only if the readers find it useful.

Chinmoy K Maity
April 2004

Acknowledgements

Writing a book like this is not usually a single author's job, especially for someone, like me, who is by no standard an expert in any of the fields covered in this book. I had to depend on a huge amount of literature written by many authors, who are experts in their respective fields. I acknowledge and express my heartfelt gratitude to them all. I also acknowledge my indebtedness to the General Medical Council (GMC), Department of Health (DH), Royal College of Physicians of London (RCPL) and Driver and Vehicle Licensing Agency (DVLA) for allowing me to use various bits and pieces from their websites in this book.

I would particularly like to acknowledge the support of my two senior nursing colleagues from Leighton Hospital, in writing the 'Medico-social issues' and 'Financial decisions' chapters: Karen Yardley, Community Liaison Manager, and Gill Sidney, Leader of Older People's Mental Health Liaison Service.

I must express my gratitude to many of my friends, colleagues and reviewers of the first edition of the book for their constructive criticism and suggestions.

I conceived the ideas arising mainly from my own needs and collected information from various sources, but obviously I expressed them the way I perceived them. Being the sole author of the book, the responsibility for any inaccuracy is mine alone.

I convey my sincere thanks to Dr Jeremy R Playfer for writing the foreword to this book.

Finally, I must thank my family, especially my two little darlings, for sparing me the time and space to complete this work.

Dedication

To Sreya, Titli and Olie
for the gift of our small world of happiness.

Section 1: Medical interviews

- Background preparation
- Presentation and common questions asked
- Current issues in the NHS, UK

Chapter 1

Background preparation

Introduction

Medical interviews are part and parcel of our professional life and we all have to face this, one of the most nerve-racking experiences, when we move up the career ladder. Like in many other aspects of life, a certain amount of planning and preparation well in advance can make these experiences less daunting or even enjoyable.

It is quite understandable that the extent and depth of preparation for an interview and the type of questions asked in an interview vary greatly at different levels of our career ladder from pre-registration house officer (PRHO) to a new consultant post. However, the basic format remains the same.

Basic principles

Medical interviews are usually organised by the personnel department (medical personnel) in the hospitals or deaneries. It is a lengthy process, which consists of:

- designing the application form, person specification and job description
- advertising the job in relevant vacancy bulletin or professional journals (e.g. *BMJ Careers*, *Hospital Doctor*, etc.)
- formation of shortlisting committee and shortlisting criteria
- formation of appointing committee (interview panel) and
- conducting the actual interview, offering job to the successful candidate and feedback to others.

Although understanding every detail of this process is not necessary for an interview candidate, a brief overview of the process is definitely helpful.

Person specification and job description: it is very important to go through the person specification and job description in detail prior to filling in an application form. *It will help you to know whether the job fits you or you fit the job. Person specification* includes the attributes required for a particular job and is based around the General Medical Council's (GMC) document *Good Medical Practice*. It has *essential* and *desirable* criteria and is based on *qualifications, knowledge and skills* (clinical, technical and communicative), *clinical and non-clinical experience* (audit, research, publication, teaching and management) and *personality* (motivation, ability to cope with stressful situations and leadership qualities). Many hospitals and deaneries have now designed a *scoring system* for shortlisting based on the above criteria.

The *shortlisting committee* is usually formed by relevant consultants under whom the successful candidates will work/rotate. In the case of the specialist registrar training programme the shortlisting committee is led by the speciality programme director. In the case of a consultant post this includes the relevant sub-speciality lead clinician, clinical director, medical director and chief executive.

The *interview panel*: in the case of PRHO and SHO (senior house officer) interviews the *interview panel* consists of the shortlisting committee and a representative from medical personnel. In the case of a specialist registrar or consultant interview the panel also includes a *chairman* who is usually a lay (non-medical) person and representatives from the relevant *Royal College* (regional advisor), *university* and *deanery*. Information about the interview panel members prior to interview may sometimes be very helpful for the candidates to prepare answers to some atypical/difficult (but some panel member's favourite) questions.

Feedback session: candidates unsuccessful either at the shortlisting or interview stage should be notified formally in writing of the result of their application as soon as a decision is made and that letter should point out the availability of feedback and counselling. A good *feedback session* is beneficial to the unsuccessful candidates for future interviews. Feedback should be given (not necessarily immediately after the interview) in a structured way and linked to an offer of career counselling.[1]

Although interviews are not foolproof ways of getting the best person for the post, they are still the core methods of selection, so making every effort to perform well in this is a very practical and sensible thing to do.

The background preparation should start long before considering applying for a job. The main aim of this lengthy preparation for a job interview is to learn the art of *'how to sell yourself in a positive light in relation to the post without over-blowing your own trumpet and sounding arrogant or big headed'*. It is a difficult job and the first step in this process is obviously to write a good curriculum vitae (CV).[2–5]

Writing a standard curriculum vitae

The very first thing you have to consider before applying for a job is writing a standard CV. In an ideal situation a CV should not be the only criterion for initial shortlisting of a candidate. Unfortunately this is the case in the United Kingdom where no other criteria, like scores in a qualifying/entrance examination, are used to assist initial shortlisting of an applicant. A CV is thus the very first self-marketing tool, which has only a few seconds to make an impact and inspire the reader's interest in you. Although the actual content of the CV is the final determinant for selection for an interview, you must make every effort to improve the presentation of your CV to create a good first impression. The following are a few practical points to remember in this regard:

- Keep it short and simple.
- Make a nice layout with wide margins and neat printing.
- Use good quality bright white paper.
- Use a good quality printer (e.g. laser printer).
- Check repeatedly for and correct spelling mistakes.
- Write the text with a positive attitude.
- Avoid too much underlining.

The contents of a CV vary and increase with progression along the career pathway. There is a basic format of a CV, but there is no hard and fast rule to follow any particular order or sequence in writing up the information. Although most hospitals have their own application forms for job applications nowadays, they also want a copy/copies of the CV along with the application form. You have to update your CV regularly and may have to edit your CV according to the needs of different applications. Never send an old CV that was intended for a different purpose. A standard good CV should include the following details:

- *Cover page* – it should contain your full name, qualifications, the job applied for with job reference number.
- *Personal details* – which include your full name, correspondence address, sex, date of birth, marital status, nationality, GMC registration type and number (if you have one) and Medical Defence Union or Medical Protection Society membership number (if you have one), etc.
- *Professional qualifications* – you must list these in chronological order, putting the most current one first. You have to mention the years of qualifications and also the names of the professional bodies awarding the degrees.
- *Academic awards and distinctions* – you can list them ever since your school level, again chronologically starting with the most recent one first.
- *Present appointment* – it should include your grade, name and address of the department and hospital, name of your educational supervisor and the duration of your contract with the starting and finishing dates.
- *Previous appointments* – all previous appointments should be listed chronologically, starting with the most recent one first, and must include the details mentioned under the present appointment.
- *Clinical experience and skills* – here you should mention briefly the experience and skills acquired from your previous jobs. You must mention your level of expertise in performing the practical procedures (supervised and unsupervised), particularly those required at your level. If you are applying for a specialist registrar post in some speciality, you can list the number of speciality-specific procedures (e.g. echocardiogram, bronchoscopy, colonoscopy, etc.) you have performed with and without supervision under a separate heading.
- *Academic (non-clinical) experience and skills* – include your experience and skills in teaching, presentations, audits, research, publications and information technology (IT). You should mention these under separate headings with a brief description of your achievements in each field starting with the most recent ones first.
- *Management experience and administrative skills* – here you should mention your leadership skill, organisational skill and communication skill under separate headings and these may not be related to your professional activity.
- *Courses attended* – list the relevant courses you have attended in chronological order with the most recent one first and you should mention any particular expertise or skill you gained from them.
- *Hobbies and interests* – mention the main ones, especially one with some significant achievement and be ready to answer confidently if you are asked any question on that topic.
- *Personality* – it is very important to mention that you are *well motivated* to do

the type of job you have applied for, you have the *ability to cope with stressful situations* and have the necessary *leadership qualities*. You may mention some examples.

- *Membership of learned societies* – include membership of learned societies like the British Medical Association (BMA), Royal College of Physicians (RCP), societies for different specialities, etc.
- *Career aspirations* – here you should write your short- and long-term future career plans with a positive attitude.
- *Referees* – you have to give the names, addresses and contact telephone and fax numbers of two to four referees, of whom at least one should be from your current job. You must ask permission from them beforehand for taking their names as referees and let them know what job you will be using their name for. If you have not met your referees for a long time, then send (them) a copy of your updated CV for their files. Do not forget to let them know when you get the job and thank them for acting as your referees.

How to improve your CV

You must always try to improve your CV to increase your chance of being shortlisted for the interview for your preferred post. The following few tips might help you in this respect.

- *Attending courses* – attending and having certificates of some courses like ALERT (acute life-threatening events recognition and treatment), BLS (basic life support), ALS (advanced life support), some speciality-based courses (e.g. postgraduate gastroenterology course, endoscopy course, echocardiography course, etc.) and courses on statistics and management will improve your chance of being shortlisted.
- *Having additional/higher degrees* – like BSc, Part 1 or full membership diploma or MD may be beneficial.
- *Having management experience* – like attending a management course, being president of a students' union or junior doctors' mess, leading a sports/cultural team in your locality/school/college/university, etc.
- *Presentations* – presentations in departmental journal club meetings, hospital grand rounds and especially in the regional, national or international meetings are very important.
- *Participating in audit* – is very important in this era of evidence-based medicine. You must participate in your departmental audits and be aware of your particular role played in the study.
- *Research and publication* – if you have one, that will definitely help you, especially if that work is relevant to your next job. However, as a HO (house officer) or SHO with a very busy work schedule and preparations for membership examination it is very difficult to have a research study or publication. To a great extent it depends on the interests of your supervising consultants. However, always be on the look out for a good/rare case for a possible *case report* and discuss your intention with your consultant.

Final preparation

- You must fill in the application form by following the instructions precisely and prepare your answers as per the *person specification* for the particular job. Before attending the interview you must get a clear view of the post you applied for. You will get most of the relevant information from the job description and discussion with the departmental secretary, medical personnel and the person currently working in that post. It will be worthwhile discussing the post with the consultant concerned and even better to arrange a departmental visit, especially if it is a long-term rotation job or a permanent job. You can get further information from the organisation's website.
- You should know your own CV inside out. Make sure you know yourself, your skills and experience, your strong and weak points and a defined career plan. Practise this several times in front of a senior colleague to make sure that you can articulate fluently, comfortably and confidently.[6]
- You should be aware of all the current hot topics in your speciality and also the important topical health-related issues. Apart from some questions to judge your professional knowledge and competency in the respective speciality, there are only a limited number of questions you can be asked in the interview. You should be aware of these common questions and prepare appropriate answers well in advance (these are discussed in the next chapters).[7,8]
- If you are attending an interview for a new consultant post, you will need some special preparation, because consultant interviews are different due to a variety of reasons:
  - the role and responsibility of a consultant are much more than those of any other post down the ladder
  - the post is going to last for a few decades, not months. You will probably spend more time with your colleagues than with your family, so it is imperative that you can work well and get on with colleagues
  - there will be a lot of extra pressure on you and your family on taking up this new role in your life, due to lifestyle changes, moving house and settling in a new area away from local friends and support networks, changing children's school, etc. You must be well aware of all these and start mental preparation well in advance.

Attending one of the *consultant interview courses* (e.g. www.medicalcommunicationskills.com, www.firstcourse-medical.co.uk, etc.) may be very helpful. You must be fully aware of all the current health-related *government policies* (e.g. revalidation, new consultant contracts, primary care trust, intermediate care, European Working Time Directive, professionalism, patient involvement unit, etc.), *political issues* and *National Service Frameworks (NSFs)* (a good source of information is www.dh.gov.uk).

- You should visit the hospital, even pre-application or pre-shortlisting informal visit, and discuss its current policies, future plans and any particular problems with the chief executive, medical director, relevant clinical director, the lead consultant, directorate manager, colleagues and ward managers. You must read the annual report of the trust, look at the hospital star rating, financial status, any current publicity, etc.

- You must spend some time, preferably along with your family, to check out the locality for houses, schools, access to motorways, entertainment facilities, etc. You may get some of this information from the internet search.[9,10]

References

1 NHS Executive (1998) *A Guide to Specialist Registrar Training*. NHSE, Leeds.
2 Majekodunmi O (2002) Sell yourself. *Hospital Doctor*. 23 March.
3 Reece D (ed.) (1995) *How to Do It* (3e). BMJ Publishing Group, London.
4 Ariyasena H, Tewari N and Livesley PJ (2005) The search for the perfect CV. *BMJ Careers*. 15 October. **331**: 167.
5 Agha R (2005) *Making Sense of Your Medical Career: your strategic guide to success* (1e). Hodder Arnold, London.
6 Camm J (2001) How role-playing exercises can enhance a job interview. *Hospital Doctor*. 7 June.
7 Persaud R (2002) Question time. *Hospital Doctor*. 9 May and 6 June.
8 Mumford CJ (2005) *The Medical Job Interviews: secrets for success* (2e). Blackwell Publishing, Oxford.
9 Various (2005) Surviving job interviews. *BMJ Careers*. 13 August. **331**: 65–80.
10 Ewies A (2001) How to prepare for your first consultant interview. *Hospital Doctor*. 22 March.

Chapter 2

Presentation and common questions asked

Presentation

When you present yourself before the interview panel, you must make sure that you look like a true professional. The following tips may help you in this regard.

- Plan your journey in advance so that you can reach your interview centre well before your interview time.
- Dress yourself in conventional and sober wear.
- Try to keep yourself as calm as possible.
- Listen to the questions carefully and, if necessary, ask them to repeat the question (not frequently).
- Try to avoid too much gesture.
- Keep eye contact with the interviewer and at times the other panel members while answering questions.
- Do not argue too much with the interviewer on any controversial topics.
- Do not forget to say 'thank you' before leaving the interview room.
- Try to stay in the interview centre till the end to accept a job offer or feedback, unless you are advised to leave earlier or you have an urgent need to go. You must inform the medical personnel in the interview panel in advance if you have to leave for any urgent need (e.g. on-call duty).[1]

If you have to give a *five/ten-minute presentation* on a particular topic to the interview panel, remember the following few points for a successful presentation.[2]

- *Less is usually more* – include a few essential key points to provide a clear and coherent coverage of a known topic. Avoid unnecessary details.
- *Keep each slide simple* – five or six bullet-points per slide is usually sufficient. Each bullet-point needs to encapsulate a particular point, which you can explain in your speech.
- *Avoid high-tech tricks* – try to keep your presentation simple, avoiding too many audiovisual effects. Always anticipate technical faults and be prepared to overcome them. Keep a back-up of paper copies and transparencies, which acts as a life-saver.
- *Watch where you stand* – avoid turning your back to the audience. Whatever mode of presentation (computer or overhead) you use, always keep a paper copy at hand to avoid reading from the screen.
- *Keep to time* – you must finish your talk within time, otherwise you will lose marks. Practising and timing your talk for a few times before the presentation will help you to get it right.

- *Question and answer time* – you must prepare yourself well to answer the post-presentation questions stemming from your talk. You have to think about the possible questions and well-argued answers. You can discuss these with your colleagues for their views, which might be of great help.

Common questions asked

The following common questions are asked in interviews to judge you as an individual professional, as a colleague team member and a colleague team leader and organiser. The interviewers do not have any interest in your personal details, which are irrelevant to the job. They are trying to select a colleague who is honest, reliable, hard-working, flexible, knowledgeable and up to date in his or her field and level.[3]

What makes you special?
Tell us a little about yourself.
This is a very common question to start with, in an interview. You should anticipate this type of question and prepare the answer. Do not reveal your personal details that are at best irrelevant to the job. Your answer should have a kind of past–present–future structure to link you and your past experiences to the job you are being interviewed for. You can begin with a brief background, starting even before you went to medical school; then discuss your experiences gained in previous jobs including your key achievements, particularly those strongly related to your current interest; and finally you should briefly give your plan for future career development, in a way that suits the position you applied for.

What are your hobbies and interests?
With this question the interviewer is trying to find out a little more about you, especially your energy and enthusiasm, morality, organisational skills and achievements outside your profession, i.e. to see whether you have a healthy balance in your life. Participating in regular sports, organising on-call rotas, organising tours (expeditions, picnics, etc.), doing voluntary work for charity and creative writing are some examples of good hobbies and interests which are worth mentioning. If the interviewer has an interest in some particular sport or current event, he/she might ask you a question on that topic, e.g. 'What is your view about the performance of the England cricket team in the recent world cup series?'

Tell us about your previous colleagues or consultants.
The interviewer is again trying to unfold some other aspects of your character relevant to the job. Do not complain in any way about any of your previous colleagues or bosses, as this will never help you. However, you should not be too positive about your previous boss or job that is very different from the post you are now applying for. A reasonable way to answer this question is to describe how your previous job and colleagues assisted you in growing to become a better candidate than before. An account of any particular experience or achievement from your previous job is worth mentioning here.

If you could change one aspect of your personality, what would it be?
What is your worst quality?

The answer to this question should focus on your self-awareness, your ability to take constructive criticism and feedback, and the ability to change yourself accordingly. Three types of bad qualities or weaknesses can be mentioned safely: first, weaknesses that are entirely irrelevant to the job; second, weaknesses that everybody has, as long as your one is not worse than others; third, the weaknesses you had in the past and have been able to cure with a positive attitude. For example: you are very approachable and cannot say 'no' to others; you are a bit overprotective; when you are busy and tired, you sometimes forget the need to take a short break and food and drink; your habit of procrastinating a bit in the past before getting down to examine a patient, but you have corrected that since.

What is the worst mistake or failure you have had in your career?

When answering this question you must remember that this is an interview, not your confessional session, and the art of winning this game lies in learning how to turn every question to your advantage. The best approach here is to admit to a mistake that has absolutely no implications for the job itself or a weakness that everyone would admit to.

Why have you changed your mind about your career?

You must anticipate this question and prepare a suitable answer if you are going to attend an interview for a job in a speciality which is different from your previous speciality. Changes in career direction are common in medicine due to a variety of reasons. Do not feel embarrassed about your change in career direction; you should put forward the change as a 'development' rather than a 'mistake'. You must be confident in answering this question, but not defensive. Emphasise how much better this new career path fits with your strengths and interests than the previous direction you were taking. You should not forget to mention how the skills you acquired in your previous job will be helpful in your new career direction.

   We should not forget a few fundamental facts of life. Life is unpredictable and, in a broader sense, nothing is a waste in life. Every bit of experience, even that of a period of unemployment, is valuable if we know how to use it. Our professional life is just a part of our whole life and our personal, social and family life is in no way less important than our professional life. You may be a very successful person as a complete human being, even though your professional career did not follow a traditionally accepted format for a while. Keeping these facts in mind will help you to answer this question more confidently.

Where do you see yourself in five years' time?

The main thing to remember here is that the interviewers want someone who is confident, ambitious and has an endless appetite for the kind of things they are interested in. The key to success in medicine is endless forward movement and the interviewers will not want someone who is going to be stagnant for five years. However, it is better to start humbly by saying that what happens in five years will depend on your performance in this job and the feedback you get. Make your long-term goal fit the job, but do not make the classic error of forcing the job to fit your deeper ambitions. Do not express any unrealistic expectation and do not aim to be somewhere further up the career ladder very much sooner than most previous incumbents have made it.

What are the duties and responsibilities of a good doctor?
If you are ill, what will you expect from your doctor?
The answer to this question should be based on the GMC's handbook on *Good Medical Practice*, which every GMC-registered doctor is expected to read and follow.[4]

'Patients must be able to trust doctors with their lives and well-being. To justify that trust, we as a profession have a duty to maintain a good standard of practice and care and to show respect for human life without any discrimination. You must always be prepared to justify your action to them. In particular as a doctor you must:

- make the care of your patient your first concern
- treat every patient politely and considerately
- respect patients' dignity and privacy
- listen to patients and respect their views
- give patients information in a way they can understand
- respect the rights of patients to be fully involved in decisions about their care
- keep your professional knowledge and skills up to date
- recognise the limits of your professional competence
- be honest and trustworthy
- respect and protect confidential information
- make sure that your personal beliefs do not prejudice patients' care
- act quickly to protect patients from risk if you have good reason to believe that you or a colleague may not be fit to practise
- avoid abusing your position as a doctor and
- work with colleagues in the ways that best serve patients' interests.'

How are you going to break bad news to the patient or patient's relatives?
This is a very common and important question, asked mainly in PRHO and SHO interviews, to assess your communication skill. Communication plays a most important role in our everyday practice and it may be between colleagues, doctor and nurse, doctor and patient, or doctor and patient's relatives. This communication may relate to a wide range of issues, starting from general discussion about the patient's problems and updating a management plan to breaking bad news like that of a serious underlying diagnosis or even death. Lack of good communication remains at the heart of most complaints and litigation.

Good communication skill is an art which we all have to learn and as we all know 'practice makes a man perfect'. Most NHS (National Health Service) hospitals and deaneries run courses on communication skills and breaking bad news, which are very useful. Further information is available from the website: www.breakingbadnews.co.uk.

However, the following are a few important practical points to consider in the context of breaking bad news to the patient and/or relatives.[5,6]

- Do not forget the key principles of *good medical practice*, i.e. respect the patient's dignity, autonomy and confidentiality.
- Where appropriate, take the patient's permission before discussing his/her care with relatives. Allow the patient, if they wish, to bring someone with them (e.g. next of kin/friend) during breaking bad news, as the patient may be upset with the bad news and may not grasp the important message from the

discussion, and this accompanying person can be of great help in this situation.

- Try to bring with you a member of the ward staff, who can stay afterwards and explain or reinforce anything you said or give emotional support.
- You must be fully aware of all aspects of the patient's management: you must go over the case notes and consult other team members, especially nursing staff, to remind yourself exactly what has happened, what is happening now and what is going to happen. This will help safeguard you from giving incorrect information, which can cause problems later on.
- Before breaking bad news you must make sure that every possible effort been made to reconfirm the diagnosis (e.g. retesting, discussion with senior colleagues or an appropriate specialist). Give them an early warning to prepare them mentally by saying, 'I am afraid the news/result is not good'.
- Make sure that the discussion takes place in a suitable environment, ideally in a quiet side room or office where you won't be disturbed.
- Be polite and patient and try to understand and feel the emotional stress they are going through.
- Be honest and do not stray from the facts. Do not feel shy to admit your ignorance, but offer to find out things you do not know.
- Explain the facts clearly in simple language, avoiding medical jargon.
- Allow time for the patient or relatives to ask questions. Make arrangements for further discussion, follow-up or counselling services, if necessary.
- Record the discussion in detail in the patient's notes with date and time.

How will you triage patients?

This question is usually asked in an interview for a SHO or registrar job, especially in an A&E (accident and emergency) or acute admission unit set-up, to assess your ability to prioritise patients' management according to need and availability of necessary resources. Usually a hypothetical situation is created in relation to this question.

Here is *an actual question* asked of one of my junior colleagues in an interview for SHO medical rotation involving A&E:

> *You are the medical SHO on call at night. Your registrar is busy managing a poorly patient in the intensive care unit and most of the A&E staff are busy attending the victims of a serious road traffic accident (RTA). You are called from the A&E resuscitation room to attend three poorly patients, all arrived at the same time:*
>
> *1   a 55-year-old male with acute severe central chest pain*
> *2   a 20-year-old girl with an attack of acute severe asthma and*
> *3   a 3-year-old floppy child who just stopped breathing.*
> *How will you manage these cases?*

To answer this type of question you have to follow the ABCDE (Airway/Breathing/Circulation/Degree or level of consciousness [AVPU (*Alert*/responds to *Vocal* stimuli/responds only to *Painful* stimuli/*Unresponsive* to all stimuli)]/Exposure [external examination]) algorithm to prioritise patients, to use all available manpower and resources and to call appropriate people for further help. A rational answer to the above question would be as follows:

> *For all practical purposes this is a hypothetical situation. All three patients need urgent attention and I hope I have at least one nursing staff to attend each of these three poorly patients. Obviously I will attend the floppy child first to start active*

resuscitation. However, I will ask one of the staff to make an arrest call so that the paediatric registrar on call comes urgently to help managing the child. I will also ask one nursing staff to be with each of the other two ill patients, to monitor their vital signs, arrange basic investigations (e.g. electrocardiogram, chest X-ray, etc.) and give urgent life-saving treatments (e.g. high-flow oxygen, glyceryltrinitrate spray, nebulised bronchodilators, etc.).

What do you think about the roles of specialist nurses?

You can expect this question in an interview for a job in a speciality where specialist nurses play a significant role (e.g. specialist nurses in diabetes, heart failure, asthma/COPD (chronic obstructive pulmonary disease), Parkinson's disease, epilepsy, urology, stoma care, etc.). They play a significant role in the management of chronic medical/surgical problems which need long-term or lifelong care and supervision in the community as well as by the specialists in the hospital. They work as an important link between patients in the community and specialist doctors in hospitals and their role is beneficial for:

- better continuity of patients' care
- better patient–professional relationship
- proven cost-effectiveness and
- reducing the specialist doctors' workload and waiting time in hospitals.

What makes you a good educator/researcher/clinician/consultant?

This is a relatively common question asked in an interview for specialist registrar or consultant posts. As we all know, some of us are natural born teachers and leaders, but most of us have to learn these qualities through proper training and practice. The most important factors common to a successful educator/researcher/clinician/consultant are *good leadership qualities*:

- motivated and enthusiastic
- committed, energetic and sensible
- knowledgeable, up to date and imaginative
- well organised, decisive and consistent
- a source of inspiration, not only information
- practical and problem-based, not a theoretician
- a good communicator
- patient and a good listener
- the ability to identify the need (e.g. of a trainee) and guide appropriately
- the ability to set an example and play a role-model
- a good sense of humour.

How are you going to make a business plan for a new service you would like to launch in your department?

This type of question is expected in an interview for a research post or a new consultant post. The intention behind the question is to judge your management and organising power. When answering this question, you have to mention the *functions* of the proposed service, necessary *workforce*, *space* and *equipment* and a *budget proposal.*[7] The steps in writing a business plan are as follows:

- Identify the need for a new service (a clinic or an investigation set up).
- Assess the extent of the need and the population to be served.
- Estimate the necessary resources and manpower.

- Describe the likely costing for the initial set-up and subsequent maintenance of the service.
- Suggest a possible source of funding, if applicable.
- Describe the project milestones in a stepwise sequence.
- Mention the potential benefits to the trust.

How will you deal with one of your poorly performing colleagues?

This is a very important question, especially in a consultant's interview, to assess your administrative quality and to explore particular aspects of your character – your interpersonal relationships and your role as a colleague team leader. The interviewers are trying to find someone who is friendly, sympathetic and helpful to his or her colleagues, but at the same time is not ready to put the patient's safety at risk or compromise the standard of care. An ideal answer to the question will be to deal with the issue in a stepwise manner and confidently as follows:

- Arrange a formal meeting with the concerned colleague in a friendly atmosphere to assess the situation and to explore any concern, worry, limitation or deficiency on his/her part.
- Advise him/her accordingly and organise further training if indicated.
- Arrange a further meeting after a specified time period to reassess the situation; this may be included in the annual appraisal process.
- However, if he/she fails to improve even after several assessments or if his/her poor performance is serious enough to put patients' safety at risk or is a criminal offence, then you have to bring it to the notice of your higher authority (e.g. clinical director, medical director or the chief executive) for further action.

How will you deal with a complaint?
How are complaints dealt with in the NHS trusts?

In a democratic society we all have the right to complain against any public service authority and the NHS is no exception to that. A complaint can be made by a patient, the patient's relatives or any NHS employee and complaints may be related to adverse events, malpractice or job-related accidents.

The most effective ways of dealing with a complaint are as follows:

- Developing an effective clinical risk management strategy which will help to prevent any major complaint arising in the first place. Users' (e.g. patients') satisfaction surveys and their suggestions about ways to improve care and service are important steps in this regard.
- Effective handling of a complaint from the very beginning – good communication skills and team working are the key to success here. While dealing with a complaint we have to keep one goal in mind – to resolve the issue in a positive way that preserves our relationship with our patient, gives us peace of mind that we handled the situation in a dignified manner and frees up our mind and our time for more positive and productive activities. A few practical tips to success:
  - do not mirror the patient's tone of voice if he or she is upset or angry, which only escalates the conflict
  - choose a quiet area to discuss with the patient/relatives, so that you are not interrupted
  - listen – let the patient/relative speak his/her mind without interruption

- avoid rationalising
- show your understanding by expressing your own feeling in a similar situation
- take action to prevent a similar situation arising in future
- assure them of an ongoing relationship.[8]

However, in spite of all these efforts on our side, we will not be able to prevent or deal with all complaints. A small number of complaints will have to be dealt with in the way described below.

The first point of contact in the complaint procedure in NHS trusts is the *Patient Advice and Liaison Service (PALS) office*, and the *patient service officer (PSO)* receives the complaint letter from the concerned party. The PSO then sends the copy of the complaint letter to the relevant clinician or manager for explanation. The PSO usually arranges a meeting with the concerned party to listen to them and explain the events in detail. The relevant clinician or the manager is usually present in this meeting to clarify the incident.

However, if the concerned party is not happy with the decision and action taken, they may request a review by the *independent review panel*. Now the trust's *complaints convenor* reviews the complaint and decides to refer the case to either an *independent expert's review* or an *independent review panel*. An independent review panel consists of three responsible citizens, usually retired persons. However, depending on the nature of the complaint the panel may have expert members.

If the concerned party is still not happy with the decision even after the independent review, they may ask for a review by the *ombudsman* or go for litigation straight away. The ombudsman is an official from an independent external agency appointed to investigate complaints against public authorities. If the ombudsman's decision does not satisfy the concerned party, they may go for litigation.

Once the complaint is considered for *litigation*, it can be settled *out of court* with the agreement of both parties or may go to *court* for a settlement.

The pathway for a complaint management is shown in Figure 2.1.

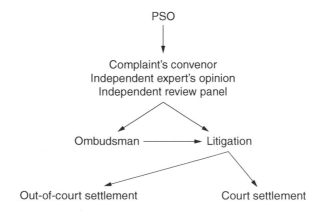

Figure 2.1 Pathway for a complaint management.

Do you have any questions?
Is there anything you want to ask the panel?
This is usually the last question in an interview session. If everything went very smoothly so far, you may finish by answering, 'No, I asked everything I needed to know already'. A better approach would be to ask a question that will reveal your interest in the post or the department. Examples include enquiring about the career progression of your predecessors or how the department is planning to cope with the new European working hours regulations, etc. However, do not waste the interviewers' valuable time by asking a trivial question, which could have been answered by the hospital porter or the medical secretary organising the interviews.

Some other common questions
It is worth preparing some ready-made answers for these in advance.

- Why did you choose the medical profession as your career?
- How do you know that you want to do medicine (or any other speciality you are being interviewed for) for the rest of your career?
- What are your strong points/weak points?
- What is your proudest achievement to date? (Sometimes the interviewer is looking for someone who is well rounded and wanting to hear that the achievement is not related to your professional work.)
- What is your source of knowledge/learning? (Interviewers often like the interviewee to include patients as a source of learning and you should not forget to mention this here.)
- Do you have any publications or presentations? If not, why?
- Have you participated in any audit? If yes, then what was your actual contribution to that study?
- Tell us about the duties and responsibilities in your current post.
- What do you specifically want to get from this job?
- If you get the job, what can the department/hospital expect from you? Or why should we give you this job?
- Are you prepared to take the extra pressure and responsibility involved in the next step of your career ladder (i.e. in the new job)?
- Can you tell us about a particular case that you managed very successfully and with great satisfaction?
- Tell us about a case that you did not manage well and learnt a lesson from.
- Can you tell us about an interesting case where you learnt a lot? Or can you tell us about an interesting case from your reflective diary? (*Reflective diaries* are usually maintained by house officers and medical students.) An interesting case does not necessarily mean a rare/interesting medical problem. Management of a particular patient, which reveals your good communication skills, good interpersonal relationships and awareness of your own limitations, will be an ideal example to mention here.
- How can you improve PRHO/SHO teaching in your hospital? (An original question was: 'Tomorrow the Dean is visiting your hospital. What suggestions you can give him to improve SHO teaching in your hospital?')
- Tell us about the most recent paper you have read that will change your clinical practice.

- Have you worked in a multidisciplinary team? What is your view about the multidisciplinary approach in patients' management?
- Give an example of where teamwork has worked well for you.
- When was the last time you called your consultant during on-call?
- How do you achieve a work/life balance?
- How do you cope with stress/criticism and complaints against you?
- Tell us about an incident/situation that challenged your professional integrity. (Here you have to mention an incident/situation where you had to sacrifice your own personal interest for the interest or safety of the patient.)
- Tell us about a situation where your own interest will take priority over that of the patient. (This will include a situation where your own safety will be at risk.)
- How do you keep up to date? (Do not forget to mention attending hospital/ departmental meetings and teaching sessions and discussion with colleagues along with reading relevant books, journals and different internet databases like Medline, Pubmed, Embase, CINAHL, etc.)
- What makes you tick (drive)?
- What non-medical book did you read lately?
- What are the NSF standards in your field/speciality (e.g. cardiology, respiratory medicine, geriatric medicine, etc.)?
- How do you see your department/hospital in five years' time?
- Why do you want to get a job in this particular region/hospital?
- If you were elected as the Health Minister of the country today, what major changes/improvements would you like to bring to the NHS?

Negotiation

Negotiation after accepting the job offer (but before signing any formal contract) may be very important, especially in the case of a consultant or staff grade post. You have to proceed with any negotiation very tactfully, with gentle persuasion and quiet diplomacy, so that you can achieve what you want without turning your future colleagues and managers against you. The common issues for negotiation are:

1 *Salary* – while moving up the junior hospital doctor ladder, there should be no drop in salary; the annual basic salary must be protected. During appointment to a consultant graded post you may negotiate for one to two incremental salary points, if you are more than 35 years of age or hold a higher degree (MD or PhD) or had worked as a locum consultant previously.
2 *Removal/relocation expenses* – appointing hospitals are supposed to reimburse these expenses, but you may have to negotiate this if the job is short term, especially if less than six months' duration.
3 *Job contract/job plan* – must be discussed in detail and agreed in accordance with the terms and conditions of the new consultant contract (*see* 'New consultant contract 2003' in the next chapter).
4 *Adequate office space and secretarial support* – all consultants must have a private office with adequate space, personal computer with internet access and at least one full-time secretary per full-time consultant.

The issues of salary and relocation expenses should be discussed with the senior medical personnel (and/or the chief executive) and other job related issues should be discussed with the relevant clinical director and/or the medical director. Professional organisations (e.g. the BMA) are very helpful in scrutinising proposed job contracts and their advice should be sought before signing any formal contract.[9]

References

1   Agha R (2005) *Making Sense of Your Medical Career: your strategic guide to success* (1e). Hodder Arnold, London.
2   Kirby R and Mundy T (2002) *Succeeding as a Hospital Doctor: the experts share their secrets* (2e). Health Press, Oxford.
3   Persaud R (2002) Question time. *Hospital Doctor.* 9 May and 6 June
4   General Medical Council (GMC) website: www.gmc-uk.org.
5   Rahaman M (2005) Dealing with relatives: what to say and how to say it. *Hospital Doctor.* 17 February.
6   Faulkner A (1998) *Effective Interaction With Patients* (2e). Churchill Livingstone, Edinburgh.
7   Reece D (ed.) (1995) *How to Do It* (3e). BMJ Publishing Group, London.
8   Wood D (ed.) (2004) *Communication for Doctors: how to improve patient care and minimize legal risks* (1e). Radcliffe Publishing, Oxford.
9   Mumford CJ (2005) *The Medical Job Interview: secrets for success* (2e). Blackwell Publishing, Oxford.

Chapter 3

Current issues in the NHS, UK

You must be fully aware of all important heath-related government policies and current issues in the NHS. These are very important, especially for an interview for a registrar or a new consultant post, and a few of them are discussed here briefly.

European Working Time Directive (EWTD)

The Council of the European Union produced a directive to protect the health and safety of workers in the European Union. It lays down the standard minimum requirements in relation to working hours, rest periods, annual leave and working arrangements for night workers. This directive was implemented in UK law as the *Working Time Regulations*, which took effect from 1 October 1998.

The key features of the EWTD are: an average of no more than 48 hours' work per week, 11 hours' continuous rest in 24 hours, 24 hours' continuous rest in seven days (or 48 hours in 14 days), 20 minutes' break in work periods of over six hours, four weeks' annual leave and for night workers an average of no more than eight hours' work in 24 hours over the reference period.

The EWTD applied to all workers with a few exceptions, including doctors in training until now. From 1 August 2004 it was extended to apply to doctors in training as a legal requirement and also as a part of the wider aims to improve the work/life balance for NHS employees. However, the provisions will be phased in with a maximum hours requirement reducing from 58 hours in 2004 to 48 hours in 2009.

The British government has applied a *derogation*, which means that it is possible for a junior doctor to work more than 13 hours in a single shift, as long as those hours are not excessive and are compensated immediately to ensure a subsequent minimum of 11 hours' rest period.[1]

Modernising Medical Careers (MMC)

It is well appreciated that implementation of the EWTD will affect the work pattern of doctors in training and will indeed challenge us to look at the way we deliver training. It has led to a disruption of the traditional hospital 'firm' structure, changing forever the relationship between a trainee and their trainer. That is why the government launched its Modernising Medical Careers strategy in February 2003 for a thorough review of the training systems and methods as well as looking at the end product of training.

> *MMC is certainly about ensuring that tomorrow's doctors are fit for purpose, but it should also secure systems that allow clinical staff to be appropriately trained and professionally developed.*[2]

In the early 1990s the Chief Medical Officer (CMO), Sir Kenneth Calman, set the task of reorganising postgraduate education for junior doctors. He asked various colleges to produce a curriculum and after long discussion the Calman team produced the recommendations for each speciality, which is known as the Calman Report. The Calman reforms brought significant changes in registrar grade training by amalgamating registrars and senior registrars into specialist registrars (SpRs). However, the senior house officer (SHO) training has remained unchanged. This issue has been addressed by the present CMO, Sir Liam Donaldson, in his *Unfinished Business*, which was sent out for consultation with the medical profession in August 2002. Following this consultation the Department of Health (DH) released a document entitled *Modernising Medical Careers*, which proposes the introduction of *Basic Medical Training (BMT)* programmes to replace the current SHO rotation programme.

The MMC career framework is in the process of evolution and the current proposals are as follows:

1 **Undergraduate medical training** – in the Medical schools for four to six years as before.
2 **Postgraduate medical training** – will be structured as follows and progress through each stage of training through open and fair competition.
   a *Foundation training programmes (F1 and F2)* - will be delivered through a so called *Foundation school*, the administrative body formed by the collaboration of medical schools, postgraduate deaneries and healthcare providers. The current pre-registration house officer (PRHO) year will be known as F1 and the first year as an SHO will be known as F2. The F1 will include three or four-month modules rather than the traditional six months of medicine and six months of surgery. F2 is intended to give a broad base of training, with common learning goals, which include acquisition of core skills and knowledge along with those outlined in the GMC document, *Good Medical Practice*.
   b *Specialist and GP training programmes (run-through training)* – will be delivered through a *specialty/GP training school*, which is formed by a range of organisations, overseen and supported by the postgraduate deans. Successful candidates can start these programmes directly after the F2 year. Once in specialist or GP training, doctors will have the opportunity to gain a Certificate of Completion of Training (CCT), subject to satisfactory progress. Each programme will have a curriculum, agreed by the Postgraduate Medical Education and Training Board (PMETB), against which doctors in training will be assessed. The required number of years of training will vary from programme to programme. After receiving a CCT, doctors will be legally eligible for entry to the Specialist or GP Register and can then apply for an appropriate senior medical appointment. A doctor who has not completed a specialist/GP training programme may apply to the PMETB for entry to the Specialist/GP Register via Articles 11 and 14 of the General and Specialist Medical Practice (Education, Training and Qualifications) Order 2003 (*see* 'PMETB' overleaf).

c *Fixed term specialist training* - these posts will be for a fixed period, probably not more than two years. They are likely to mirror the early years of training in a specialty/GP training programme and trainees will be assessed against explicit standards.

d *Career posts* – these are service delivery posts with no formal specialty training elements. However, employers' appraisal and relevant continuing professional development will be an essential part of these doctors' careers. These posts will only be available in secondary care.

3 **Senior medical appointments** – doctors who have their name in the Specialist/GP Register (either through CCT or via Articles 11 and 14), will be eligible for these posts and include GP principals, other employed GPs, consultants or other specialist roles. Their roles will be determined by the service.

Thus 'an early foundation programme emphasizes the acquisition of clinical and professional skills followed by specialist training that is focussed on the needs of the NHS for accredited doctors. Both are designed to create a modern workforce that works effectively with other health professionals for patients'.[2]

The implementation of the EWTD and the proposed shortening of the training period envisaged within the MMC will significantly diminish the experience gained by the trainees, so the learning through clinical encounters must be optimised. The old 'apprenticeship model' learning or 'role-model' teaching can no longer be practicable or desirable. The didactic teaching should be replaced by a modern, learner-centred, enquiring, reflective and adult-style teaching. To achieve this goal we need an extension of the role of educational supervisor, improvements in career advice, counselling and mentoring and changing consultant contracts (new consultant contract).

The document *Modernising Medical Careers* also states that the *non-consultant career grades (NCCGs)*, now known as staff and associate specialists (SAS), should be aided and facilitated to acquire a CCT. A Postgraduate Medical Education and Training Board (PMETB) has been formulated to organise competency-based assessment to ensure the quality of the end product of training. It will also provide competency-based assessment (articles 11 and 14) for doctors holding a primary medical qualification in the UK or abroad to apply for direct entry to the specialist register held by the General Medical Council (GMC).

A few proposed MMC timeline targets are as follows:

- *1 August 2005:* Foundation programme to begin. The first cohort of F1 doctors started their placements all over the country.
- *1 August 2006:* The first cohort to go into their F2 year.
- *August 2006:* Application process for speciality selection training to be agreed.
- *August 2007:* The first MMC cohort to enter specialist training.[1,2]

Postgraduate Medical Education and Training Board (PMETB)

Postgraduate medical education and training in the UK have been managed until now by the *Specialist Training Authority (STA)* of the medical Royal Colleges and the *Joint Committee on Postgraduate Training for General Practice (JCPTGP)* in conjunction with NHS postgraduate deaneries and the medical Royal Colleges. It has been realised that there is a lack of uniformity of standards across the country because of variations in syllabus and different criteria set by different medical Royal Colleges.

To develop a single, unifying framework for postgraduate medical education and training across the UK, the government established the PMETB by the General and Specialist Medical Practice (Education, Training and Qualifications) Order (GSMPO), which was approved by Parliament on 4 April 2003.

The PMETB will have the statutory duty to establish, maintain and develop standards and requirements relating to postgraduate medical education and training in the UK. The PMETB is accountable to Parliament and will act independently of government as the UK competent authority. The Board comprises 25 members, of whom 17 are medical and eight lay including the Chair. A member from the SAS doctors would be appointed to each of the PMETB statutory committees: the training and assessment committees. The PMETB must fulfil responsibilities to three constituencies:

- patients and the public
- doctors in training
- employers and those commissioning services.

The PMETB took up its full statutory powers on 30 September 2005. It will continue to work in partnership with the medical Royal Colleges and faculties, and the Department of Health's MMC team in the transition period between 2005 and 2007 in the development of curricula, assessments, programmes and the national quality-assurance framework. After assuming competent authority the PMETB will have three main areas of activity:

- approval (e.g. curricula, assessments, programmes)
- certification of applicants for direct entry to the specialist register
- quality assurance and evaluation.

The Board's remit covers basic and higher specialist training but does not cover:

- undergraduate medical education, nor that of pre-registration doctors, which remain the responsibility of the GMC and universities
- undergraduate and postgraduate dental education and training, which remain the responsibility of the General Dental Council.

The *specialist register*, maintained by the GMC, is a list of all those doctors who are legally entitled to take up substantive, fixed-term or honorary consultant posts in the NHS. Since the PMETB assumed full statutory power, there are two main routes for entry into this specialist register:

- by gaining a *Certificate of Completion of Training (CCT)* or
- by obtaining a *Statement of Eligibility* for specialist registration.

The Statement of Eligibility for specialist registration is considered a 'standard of equivalence' to CCT (article 14[4]) or the knowledge and skill of a consultant in the NHS (article 14[5]). However, this Statement of Eligibility may not automatically be accepted in the European Economic Area (EEA) outside the UK, as this does not fall within European mutual recognition arrangements.

The Board is now in the process of publishing the eligibility criteria for entry into the specialist register in each speciality. The entries, re-entries, exits and flexibility in postgraduate education and training as proposed by the Board and further updates are available from the Board's website.[2,3]

New consultant contract 2003

The implementation of EWTD and MMC is going to have a huge impact on the NHS workforce planning and the role of consultants. The time required for direct clinical care, in addition to management and administrative activities, keeping up to date, training and all of the other professional activities, results in great pressure on individual consultants and the service as a whole. This demanded a change in the consultants' job contract with the aim of helping NHS organisations collaborate with the profession to support service improvement and help improve doctors' working lives.

After a long negotiation between the British Medical Association (BMA) and the Department of Health (DH), a *New Consultant Contract 2003* was finalised on 20 October 2003 and it was decided that from 31 October 2003 all new consultant posts in the NHS must be advertised in terms of the new contract.

The two main areas of changes in this new contract are:

- *changing the measure of consultants' work* – now expressed as programmed activities (PAs), each representing four hours (three hours at night/out of hours) of consultant time
- *attaching a time value to programmed activities* – 'to provide greater transparency about the level of commitment expected of consultants by the NHS'.[4]

Under the new terms and conditions, a full-time consultant will have a commitment of ten programmed activities per week. Additional programmed activities can be arranged by agreement between the consultant and the employer. However, as per NHS Pension Agency guidance, pensionable pay will include basic salary for up to ten programmed activities. Consultants participating in an on-call rota will be paid a supplement in addition to a basic salary. The level of supplement, which ranges between 1% and 8% of full-time basic salary, will depend on the consultant's rota frequency and the category of the consultant's on-call duties as follows:

- *Category A* applies where the consultant is typically required to return immediately to site when called, or has to undertake interventions with a similar level of complexity to those that would normally be carried out on site, such as telemedicine or complex telephone consultations.
- *Category B* applies where the consultant can typically respond by giving telephone advice and/or by returning to work later. (*See* Table 3.1.)

Table 3.1 Level of supplement for on-call availability

| Frequency of rota commitment | Value of supplement as % of full-time basic salary | |
	Category A	Category B
*High frequency:*1 in 1 to 1 in 4	8%	3%
*Medium frequency:*1 in 5 to 1 in 8	5%	2%
*Low frequency:*1 in 9 or less frequent	3%	1%

The duties and responsibilities of a consultant have been clearly explained in this new contract under two main headings:

- *Direct clinical care* – Any activity that involves the care of individual patients should be included in PAs of direct clinical care. This includes a wide range of duties: outpatient clinics, inpatient ward rounds and operations, clinic letters, reviewing and communicating results, providing advice to GPs and other healthcare practitioners, telephone consultations, seeing relatives, multidisciplinary team meetings, X-ray meetings, case conferences/presentations, prioritising referrals, organising investigations, supervising other members of the team, providing clinical reports and other clinical correspondence, addressing complaints or clinical incidents and so on. Predictable emergency work out of hours (e.g. ward rounds in the evening and weekends) and during normal working hours (e.g. post-take ward rounds) must be scheduled in the PAs separately from other clinical duties (e.g. speciality ward rounds and clinics etc.).
- *Supporting professional duties* – These are essential professional commitments, outside direct clinical care, for maintaining and improving clinical service. These duties include teaching, mentoring, self-education, audit, appraisal, clinical governance, continuing professional development (CPD), revalidation, service development and research. This also includes competency-based assessment of the trainees by direct observation – mini clinical evaluation exercise (Mini-CEX), directly observed procedural skills (DOPS) and 360-degree assessment of behaviour and interpersonal skills, or multi-source feedback (MSF). The new contract also recommends that external duties might include 'reasonable quantities of work for the Royal Colleges in the interest of the wider NHS' (national duties) (e.g. college tutor, speciality advisor, regional advisor etc.). The list is ever expanding, time-consuming and has great impact upon the time for clinical workload. All these supporting professional duties must be recognised by the employing organisations in the consultant's job plan and should have formal agreed sessional commitment.

Within a full-time framework of 10 PAs per week, it has been agreed that, in England, a full-time consultant will devote on average 7.5 PAs for direct clinical care and 2.5 PAs for supporting professional duties (in Wales this is 7 PAs and 3 PAs respectively). However, those regularly involved in various national duties for the wider NHS may need an extra 1–2 PAs for supporting professional duties and these should be included in the job plan by agreement between the consultant and employing organisation.

The Clinical Academic Consultant Contract (England) 2003 recommends that a full-time academic consultant post should have ten PAs per week, of which five involve work for the NHS and five for the university. However, this is not prescriptive and depends on the requirements of the job. The PAs for the NHS should follow a 3:1 ratio of direct clinical care to supporting professional duties. The PAs for the university should follow the BMA guidelines.[4-7]

Improving Working Lives (IWL)

IWL is another initiative from the DH and it sets out a series of performance standards for NHS employers to improve the working lives of NHS employees. The aim is to encourage employers to develop a range of policies and practices which support personal and professional development and enable employees to achieve a healthy work/life balance. An IWL accreditation kitemark will be awarded to employers who can demonstrate, via portfolios of evidence, that they are improving the working lives of their employees.

The IWL initiative aims to make clear that every person employed by the NHS can work in an organisation that is flexible, supportive and family friendly, and that has a commitment to improving diversity, tackling discrimination, harassment and bullying issues and developing the skills of its entire staff.

There are three stages of development as follows:

- *Pledge* – involves putting in place the people, policies and planning to achieve accreditation.
- *Practice* – involves reaching the standard and putting policies into practice.
- *Practice plus* – NHS employers achieving *Practice* accreditation will be reviewed by agreement between the trust and their regional IWL accreditation team to check that any gaps in the standards have been remedied. *Practice plus* accreditation will be awarded when the regional IWL accreditation team is satisfied that the standard is being met in full for all staff.

Targets to be achieved are as follows:

- *By April 2001* – all trusts have achieved Stage One (Pledge) of the IWL accreditation.
- *By April 2003* – all NHS employers are expected to be accredited as putting the IWL standard into practice.

There are various schemes that feed into the IWL initiative:

- *Flexible careers scheme (FCS)* – this is administered by NHS Professionals and the employment costs for part-time posts on the FCS are centrally funded, so trusts will be reimbursed a percentage of the cost. FCS provides scope for doctors to return to practice after a career break, or to do part-time work. All FCS posts are designed to provide sufficient medical and clinical practice for revalidation purposes.
- *Flexible training (FT) options* – this allows trainees to opt for the flexible training scheme and build up their credits towards the Certificate of Completion of Training (CCT). Flexible training is organised through postgraduate deaneries and trainees must undertake a minimum of 50% of full-time training posts in order to qualify.
- *Flexible retirement options* – this scheme encourages those consultants nearing retirement to reconsider their job roles and perhaps reduce hours and service demands without damaging their pension benefits.
- *Childcare strategies* – these aim to encourage those with children to come back to the NHS workforce. The NHS Plan outlines targets for increasing and improving childcare facilities for NHS staff.[1]

Intermediate care

The health system in the UK is run by the local health authorities and it has a two-tier system:

- community-based primary care focused on a generalist approach
- hospital-based secondary care focused on a specialist approach.

The impetus for a new type of service called *intermediate care* in the late 1990s was given a very considerable boost following the consultation on the *National Bed Inquiry* and the subsequent publication of the *NHS Plan*. An intermediate care type service will play an important role in bridging the gaps between primary and secondary care.

The NHS Plan set out a major new programme to promote independence for older people, through developing a range of services that are delivered in partnership between primary and secondary healthcare, local authority services, in particular social care, and the independent sector. One of the critical elements in this programme is to develop new intermediate care services. The NHS Plan announced an extra investment of £900 million annually by 2003/04 for inter-mediate care and related services to promote independence. The next target, to achieve by March 2004, was at least 5000 extra intermediate care beds and 220 000 people receiving intermediate care services.

Physicians have been somewhat ambivalent about intermediate care and the degree of involvement of doctors from primary and secondary care has been very variable in different parts of the country. Although intermediate care was con-ceived as an issue in all specialities, there has been very little secondary care input into intermediate care by other specialities apart from geriatric medicine. Inter-mediate care is *Standard three* in the *National Service Framework for Older People*. The aim of this standard is to provide integrated services to promote faster recovery from illness, prevent unnecessary acute hospital admissions, support timely discharge and maximise independent living.

Intermediate care has been seen as the solution to a number of different prob-lems. From a clinical viewpoint, it was seen as the re-investment in rehabilitation-type services, particularly for older people, in a properly organ-ised multidisciplinary environment, nearer to home, without the perceived dangers of prolonged in-hospital care. From a managerial perspective, such services were seen as an answer to the chronic NHS bed crisis and to ensure that the NHS Plan targets for elective surgery could be met.

However, concern has been raised that development of intermediate care reflected an ageist policy being pursued by central government. The worry was that older people were being shunted into second-rate, under-resourced services and deprived of the resources and investigations available in district general hospitals. The intermediate care scheme should have built-in clinical governance arrangements from its inception to protect against such discrimination.

A national evaluation of intermediate care has been commissioned and the result will be available in 2006.[1]

Primary care trusts (PCTs)

In the late 1990s the British government realised that the NHS was not fulfilling people's expectations and reform is the precondition for sustaining public confidence in the health service. It appreciated the public view that staff in public services have been simply doing their best inside a system that for too long has been under-resourced and by and large people trust the NHS frontline staff (doctors, nurses and other health professionals). It also realised that most of the NHS frontline staff feel that the NHS is like a centrally run bureaucracy and the NHS cannot be run from Whitehall.

With the above realisation the DH launched the *NHS Modernisation Agency* and the *NHS Plan* to reform and redesign the NHS over a decade around the needs of patients. This decade-long modernisation process involves *significant structural reorganisation* and a *huge cultural shift* in NHS healthcare delivery. The DH planned to move the centre of gravity within the health service itself from *Whitehall* to the *NHS frontline* in a phased programme to decentralise the system and put power and resources in the hands of the NHS frontline. *Shifting the Balance of Power* within the NHS is the programme of change brought about to empower frontline staff and patients in the NHS and its main feature is giving the locally based PCTs the role of running the NHS and improving health in their areas.

The structural reorganisation plan involves: demolition of the existing 99 local health authorities and possibly all eight regional offices and creation of new *strategic health authorities (SHAs)* and transfer of extra powers to *primary care trusts (PCTs)*. (PCTs are the local statutory organisations in the English NHS responsible for improving public health, providing primary healthcare, and commissioning secondary and tertiary care services for an average population of 250 000.) The proposed boundaries of the 28 new SHAs were announced and they started functioning from April 2002. Each SHA covers an average population of 1.5 million and their main function is to support the *PCTs* and the *NHS trusts* (secondary care trusts) in delivering the NHS Plan in their area. Although both NHS trusts and PCTs will be accountable to the new SHAs, both will have greater operational freedom. NHS trusts will be responsible for providing local hospital and specialist services. PCTs will be responsible for commissioning them as well as providing primary and community services.

The first 13 pioneering new PCTs were announced by the Health Minister John Denham in January 2000 and they started functioning from 1 April 2000. Local GPs and nurses see and treat 90% of all patients seen by the NHS. They oversee how patients go into hospital, care for them when they leave hospital and work with social services and other agencies to look after them at home and in the community. Therefore the PCTs will be best run by these healthcare professionals who know the needs of their patients. PCTs will play a key role in developing fast, modern and convenient health services for patients. PCTs will give local doctors, nurses and other health professionals more control over the way the NHS develops than ever before. It will give them:

- a bigger say in how NHS money is spent than ever before (the typical PCT will control over 80% of the health spending on its local population)
- new power to provide local health services such as community nursing, community hospitals and services for the elderly

- the power to work with hospital clinicians to determine how other services are provided and to enable more services to be delivered closer to patients
- new powers to work with local health authorities to improve the care of patients in the community.

All PCTs across the country started full functioning from 1 April 2004. However, over the last year it has been revealed that the PCTs failed to perform their role, especially in bringing the strategic changes in secondary care, and this has led to renewed interest in strengthening the commissioning function in the NHS. The government's new policy *Commissioning a Patient-Led NHS* is aimed at restructuring the PCTs including changes to their boundaries, *practice-based commissioning (PBC)* and cutting management costs by 15%, by outsourcing management, leadership and commissioning functions to the private sector. PBC (a scheme whereby practices are delegated a purchasing budget for their enrolled population) is supposed to be adopted by all general practices in England by the end of 2006. Changes are also taking place in secondary care with the goal of creating foundation hospitals – with the introduction of the *Independent Sector Treatment Centre (ISTC)* and *Payment by Results (PbR)* programmes, etc. Further organisational changes are expected in the near future.[1]

Medical professionalism

Medical professionalism has been defined as 'a combination of technical knowledge and skills, the upholding of strong ethical principles and values, and belief in the notion of medicine as a vocation, with the interest of the patient always paramount'.[6] Traditionally, medical professionalism is learnt by examples set by senior doctors, which can have an enduring effect, so they have a responsibility to make it the right effect.

Historically, the idea of professionalism has gone hand in hand with the concept of professional self-regulation, i.e. professionals themselves have agreed the standards that guide their professional conduct and behaviour to the potentially vulnerable individuals, the patients. However, after several high-profile cases of failure in professional self-regulation (e.g. the Bristol baby heart scandal), the professions can no longer be seen to be judge and jury in their own cause. The growth of consumerism, easier access to information, and a better educated, more demanding, less deferential public have led to the questioning of professionalism as an acceptable means on its own of safeguarding standards and reflecting the interests of those served by the professionals. The government has also recognised the need for a more objective, independent means of setting standards and judging the extent to which they have been met. To keep pace with changing times and demands, the traditional medical professionalism needs necessary changes to develop a new professionalism which will demonstrably be more sensitive to the views of patients and public.

There are numerous factors threatening medical professionalism:

- Enforced changes in work practice, particularly shift work, are leading to a loss of continuity of care and diminution of personal responsibility.
- The loss of the traditional medical team structure and associated loss of the opportunity for senior leadership by example.

- The advent of the NHS 'blame culture', rising consumerism in healthcare and the fall in public confidence in doctors, due to the high-profile failures of a few, are leading to a crisis in morale among the profession.

It is vitally important to sustain our values in the face of these factors. The RCP believes that it is necessary to redefine the concept of medical professionalism and to act in order to prevent its further erosion, and it has already started working in that direction.[6-8]

Patient Involvement Unit (PIU)

Considering service users' views when planning and improving any clinical service is an essential part of modern healthcare. The NHS Plan identified 'the involvement of public in health services in several capacities with the overall aim to give patients and the public a voice in national policy and local services' as a key issue.

Collaboration of patients, carers and the medical profession will have a powerful joint voice to bring their concerns to the attention of the government. Moreover, as experts on their illness, patients can do much to improve the quality of healthcare services and their involvement in strategies affecting care provision is essential. Keeping these in mind, the RCP established the Patient Involvement Unit (PIU) in September 2003 to promote this partnership. This unit comes under the remit of the Professional Affairs Department and it has a full-time patient involvement manager.

The main aim of the PIU is to identify areas where patients and doctors can build cooperative and mutually beneficial relationships. For better involvement of patients and the general public, the college working group recommended the creation of the following two support groups:

- *Patient and Carer Network* – This ensures that the interests of patients, carers and the wider public are fully integrated in the work of the college and helps the college develop and enhance its relationship with the users of the NHS. The network consists of approximately 75 patients, carers and members of the public who have been recruited from a range of backgrounds through adverts in the national press. Members join the network for three years and undertake a number of activities.
- *Patient and Carer Involvement Steering Group* – This provides the strategic input into the PIU and assists the development of overall college policy in respect of improving clinical standards for the benefit of patients, carers and the public. The Steering Group comprises six college staff and six lay representatives and works in close collaboration with the Patient and Carer Network.[6]

National Patient Safety Agency (NPSA)

A *patient safety incident* is defined as any unintended or unexpected incident which could have led or did lead to harm for one or more patients receiving NHS-funded care. There are an estimated 900 000 patient safety incidents in the UK per year. An expert group, led by the Chief Medical Officer, Sir Liam Donaldson, called *An Organisation with a Memory* recognised that 'there has been little systematic learning from patient safety incidents and service failure in the NHS in the past' and drew attention to the scale of the problem of potentially avoidable events that result in unintended harm to patients.[9]

In June 2000, the government accepted all the recommendations made in the report of this expert group and this formed the basis of development of the National Reporting and Learning System (NRLS) and *National Patient Safety Agency (NPSA)*. The NRLS started functioning from November 2003 and it will be implemented in stages across the NHS.

The NPSA is a *special health authority* created to coordinate the efforts of all those involved in healthcare, and more importantly to learn from adverse incidents occurring in the NHS. It is *not* a performance management, regulatory or investigative body, and is interested only in the *how* and not the *who*. The NPSA receives the information on incidents through the NRLS. The NRLS is confidential and anonymous, and does not store any identifiable details of the reporter, staff or patient involved in the patient safety incident. Staff in every NHS organisation in England and Wales will be able to report the incident to the NRLS through a specially designed electronic reporting form *(eForm)* or through their organisation's local risk-management system. It is also in the process of developing a version of the electronic reporting form for the public and relevant third parties such as the NHS Patient Advice and Liaison Services (PALS). Currently the NPSA is taking calls from the public about their healthcare experiences via a dedicated PALS.

The NPSA will play a key role in bringing patient safety to a national level, enabling the entire NHS to learn from incidents and make itself safer and more stress free for patients by:

- helping to develop an 'open and fair', more blame-free culture in the NHS
- making sure that incidents and near misses are reported by the healthcare staff in the first place
- collecting and analysing information on adverse incidents from local NHS organisations, NHS staff, patients and carers
- ensuring that, where risks are identified, work is undertaken on producing solutions to prevent harm, specify national goals and establish mechanisms to track progress.

From 1 April 2005, the NPSA's work also encompasses the following:

- safety aspects of hospital design, cleanliness and food (transferred from NHS Estates)
- ensuring safety in research, through its responsibility for the Central Office for Research Ethics Committees (COREC)
- supporting local organisations in addressing their concerns about the performance of individual doctors and dentists, through its responsibility for the National Clinical Assessment Service (NCAS)
- managing the contracts with three confidential enquiries (National Confidential Enquiry into Patient Outcome and Death [NCEPOD], Confidential Enquiry into Maternal and Child Health [CEMACH] and National Confidential Inquiry into Suicide and Homicide by people with mental illness [NCISH]), the responsibility being transferred from the National Institute for Clinical Excellence (NICE).

The NPSA's new guide to good practice, *Seven Steps to Patient Safety: the full reference guide*, details the steps that NHS organisations and teams can take to achieve safer care for all.[1,9]

References

1   Department of Health (DH) website: www.dh.gov.uk.
2   Various (2005) Symposium on Modernising Medical Careers. *Hospital Medicine*. March. **66** (3): 134–46.
3   Postgraduate Medical Education and Training Board (PMETB) website: www.pmetb.org.uk.
4   Royal College of Physicians (2004) *Guidance on the New Consultant Contract, and its Implications for Job Plans (Programmed Activities)*. Royal College of Physicians of London's website: www.rcplondon.ac.uk.
5   Department of Health (2003) *Advance Letter AL (MD) 3/2003: Introduction of the 2003 Consultant Contract (England)*. 18 December. Department of Health, London.
6   Royal College of Physicians (2005) *Consultant Physicians Working With Patients* (3e). RCP, London.
7   Black C and Craft A (on behalf of the Academy of Medical Royal Colleges) (2004) The competent doctor: a paper for discussion. *Clinical Medicine*. November/December. **4** (6): 527–33.
8   Royal College of Physicians (2004) Doctors in society: medical professionalism in a changing world. Report of a Working Party of the Royal College of Physicians. *Clinical Medicine*. **5**(6) (Suppl 1).
9   National Patient Safety Agency website: www.npsa.nhs.uk.

Section 2: Medico-legal issues

- Capacity, consent and confidentiality
- Financial decisions
- Compulsory detention and treatment
- Welfare and healthcare decisions
- Mental Capacity Bill 2004
- Medical standards of fitness to drive
- Brain death

Chapter 4

Capacity, consent and confidentiality

Introduction

With the changing society modern-day medical practice is increasingly litigation prone and the list of legal issues arising from *medical malpractice* (immoral, illegal or unethical professional conduct) or *negligence* (breach of legal duty of care, resulting in injury to the patient) is never-ending. I am not in a position to discuss all these issues here, but my intention is to give you a brief and very simplified overview of the common medico-legal issues which we have to deal with in our everyday practice.

Medicine is an international enterprise and doctors and scientists are not limited by national boundaries. Most of the medico-legal issues discussed here take place in the international arena, but the medical law and legal framework for medical practice are different in different countries. The issues discussed in this book are applicable in the United Kingdom; however, there are some differences in some legislation in Scotland and Northern Ireland from those in England and Wales (e.g. a proxy decision maker can make a decision on behalf of an incompetent adult in Scotland, but not in Northern Ireland, England and Wales).

In many areas of medical practice there is no *statute* (the written law passed by a legislative body); however, these are covered by *case law* (the law established by following the judges' decisions in previous similar cases) or *common law* (the collection of judges' decisions about the law on subjects where Parliament has not yet passed a statute).

The distribution of power and responsibility for decision making remains at the heart of most medico-legal problems. Patients' autonomy being the key principle of modern medical practice, it is a legal requirement for good practice to get valid consent from the patient in all aspects of management. Therefore the very first step in this process is to assess the patient for his/her capacity/competency to give valid consent.

Capacity/competency

Any individual above the age of 16 years is presumed to have the capacity to make a treatment decision unless proved otherwise. Patients under the age of 16 years need assessment of their mental capacity to consent for a proposed treatment. However, any refusal of a necessary treatment by a patient under the age of 18 years can be over-ruled by the court or someone with parental responsibility for the benefit of the patient.

When there is any doubt or concern about the mental capacity of the patient, it should be formally assessed by appropriate professionals. Capacity is *decision-specific* and assessment of capacity must be made in relation to a particular proposed intervention. Just because a person has dementia, learning disability or mental illness or is under 16 years of age does not necessarily mean that they are incapable of making a particular decision. The person may have the capacity to consent to some simple interventions but not to other complex ones. Capacity may be *fluctuating* over time and all such assessments must be recorded in the patient's notes. Patients' valid *advance directives* and *best interest* principles will guide his/her future management decisions.

For most day-to-day decisions there is no formal process of assessment of mental capacity. However, for more important decisions like medical treatment and legal matters, patients need formal assessment of their mental capacity to make relevant decisions. For *legal matters* such as wills or enduring power of attorney issues, a solicitor has to make the judgement about the capacity of the person to understand the nature of the transaction, but if there is any doubt they should get an opinion from a doctor or other appropriate professional. For decisions about the person's capacity in relation to *medical issues*, the physician with the primary responsibility for the patient's care is usually responsible for this assessment; however, complex cases involving difficult issues about the future health and well-being or even the life of the patient should be referred to an independent psychiatrist, ideally one approved under *section 12(2)* of the Mental Health Act. If there is still any doubt or concern about the capacity of the patient, then legal advice should be sought for applying to the High Court for a ruling.

This assessment of mental capacity includes a formal 'mental status examination' (e.g. Falstein's mini-mental state examination) to elicit information about the individual's orientation to time, place, person and situation; their mood and affect; the content of their thought and perceptions with particular regard to delusion and hallucinations; their intellectual capacity; their past history of any psychiatric illness; their recent and remote memory and logical sequencing. Assembling such information is very useful and important in determining an individual's capacity.

However, it is suggested that capacity to consent in relation to a particular treatment is made up of the following elements and a person is considered to have the capacity to make an individual decision about treatment if he/she fulfils all of them.

- *Understands the information* given to them in a clear way, using simple, non-technical language, visual aids, leaflets and signing if necessary. The information in broad terms should include the purpose and nature of the proposed intervention, the principal benefits and risks associated with it, possible alternative measures and the likely consequence of not receiving the proposed treatment.
- *Believes* and is able to weigh the information.
- *Retains* the information long enough to make a decision/choice.

Mental incapacity means that a person is either unable to make a decision because of his/her mental state, because he/she cannot communicate that decision or a combination of the two.[1-3]

Consent

Consent is a decision/agreement to an action based on knowledge of what the action involves and its likely consequences.

It is a general legal and ethical principle that valid consent must be obtained before starting treatment or physical examination or providing personal care for a patient. While there is no English statute setting out the general principles of consent, *common law* has established that touching a patient without valid consent may constitute the *civil* (claim for damages as a result of treatment) or *criminal* (assault or indecent assault) offence of battery.

Current medical case laws in the United Kingdom are based on the existing case laws of the *European Court of Human Rights*. Before making a decision the patient must know that he/she is fully entitled to enjoy the following *basic human rights*, so long as he/she is not interfering with others' rights:

- *(Article 2)* Protection of right to life – confers a right of self-determination in relation to life and death. However, any act with a primary intention of bringing about a patient's death would be unlawful, even though suicide itself has been decriminalised since 1961.
- *(Article 3)* Prohibition of torture, inhuman or degrading treatment or punishment – no one shall be subjected to torture or inhuman or degrading treatment or punishment.
- *(Article 5)* Right to liberty and security, unless under lawful detention.
- *(Article 8)* Right to respect for private and family life, home and correspondence.
- *(Article 9)* Freedom of thought, conscience and religion – everyone has the right to say 'no' or 'yes' or 'I don't know' or 'I don't understand'. They have the right to say what they feel, think or prefer and to change their mind and think differently in the future. They have the right to be different from others in their feelings, ideas, wishes, tastes, needs, standards and values and to make decisions (even mistakes) that may not meet with the approval of others.
- *(Article 12)* Right to marry and found a family according to national laws.
- *(Article 14)* Prohibition of discrimination in enjoyment of Convention rights – everyone has the right to be treated with respect, irrespective of their age, sex, sexuality, race, class, employment status or disability.

To be *valid consent* it must satisfy the following criteria:

- The patient must be competent.
- The patient must be fully informed about the proposed intervention.
- Consent must be given voluntarily without undue internal or external pressure.

The need for valid consent extends to all aspects of the relationship between a doctor and patient as follows:

- treatment of the patient
- confidentiality and disclosure of information
- research study
- screening tests
- studying and teaching
- clinical photography
- publishing.

There are two types of consent, depending on the way it is given.

- *Implied consent* – here the patient's actions/gestures tell you that they are happy for you to proceed. The classic example is when a patient rolls up a sleeve when you ask if you can take their blood pressure.
- *Express consent* – here the patient can give consent verbally or in writing. The GMC suggests that *written consent* should be taken in the following cases where:
  - the treatment or procedure is complex, or involves significant risks and/or side effects
  - there may be significant consequences for the patient's employment, social or personal life
  - the interventions are primarily done for non-therapeutic purposes (e.g. screening)
  - the treatment is part of a research programme
  - consent for storage and use of gametes and live transplant of an organ, which are legal requirements as well.

A competent person can refuse consent or can withdraw consent at any time. Once consent is given, it generally remains valid for an indefinite duration unless withdrawn by the patient. However, if consent was obtained a significant time before the intervention, it is good practice to reconfirm that, prior to the intervention, the patient is still competent.

Consent to research

Research, involving people directly or indirectly, is vital in improving the care of present and future patients and the health of the population as a whole. However, the benefits and risks to the people involved in a research study may be uncertain and unclear. The volunteers and patients should be given the fullest possible information, presented in an easy to understand way, before they consent. It is therefore vital to make sure that participants are aware of the following:

- the research is not contrary to the individual's best interests
- it is a research study and the results are unpredictable
- details of possible benefits and risks
- evidence of approval of a research ethics committee
- they can withdraw at any time
- time to read and consider the information
- no pressure to get involved.

Consent to screening

Screening healthy or asymptomatic people to detect genetic predispositions or early signs of debilitating or life-threatening conditions can be an important tool in providing effective care. However, there are a great many uncertainties and potentially serious consequences involved with the screening process, so the participants should be fully informed about the following facts before they make properly informed consent:

- the screening is not contrary to the individual's best interests
- the purpose and nature of screening

- the likelihood of positive/negative findings and possibility of false-positive/negative results
- the uncertainties and risks attached to the screening process
- any significant medical, social or financial implication of proposed screening
- follow-up plans, including availability of counselling and support services.[1,3-8]

Confidentiality

To provide good and effective care doctors need information about patients, which may be private and sensitive. Patients may be reluctant to give this information without assurance about confidentiality, which is central to the trust between doctors and patients, so doctors have an obligation to respect patients' confidentiality.

The key principles of good practice governing disclosure of confidential information about a patient are as follows:

- The patient's consent must be obtained prior to disclosure of information, wherever that is practicable.
- Anonymise data where unidentifiable data will serve the purpose.
- Keep disclosures to the minimum necessary.
- A patient's *implied consent* is enough for disclosure of information to the healthcare team to provide their care or for local clinical audit of that care.
- Keep up to date with and observe the requirements of statute and common law, including data protection legislation.
- Seek legal advice if the legal basis for a request for information is not clear.
- In the UK the common law requires *express consent* for disclosure of *identifiable data (name, address and full postcode)*, unless there is a legal provision authorising or requiring disclosure of data or an over-riding public interest in the disclosure, as in the following cases:
  - disclosures required by law, e.g. notification of a communicable disease
  - disclosure in relation to a court order
  - disclosure in the public interest, e.g. disclosures in relation to serious crime, sex offenders, drink driving, control of communicable diseases etc.
  - disclosure to protect the patient or others, e.g. disclosure to assist in the prevention, detection or prosecution of a serious crime like child abuse.

A doctor's duty of confidentiality continues even after the death of the patient, as disclosure of some confidential information may cause distress to the family and persons close to the patient. However, there are circumstances in which you have an obligation to disclose such information:

- to assist a coroner with an inquest
- to national confidential inquiries or other clinical audit or for education or research
- on the death certificate
- to those lawfully entitled to deal with the person's will or life assurance policy.[1,4,6-8]

References

1   The General Medical Council's current documents on 'Duties of a doctor'. Available at www.gmc-uk.org.

  - Good Medical Practice.
  - Confidentiality: protecting and providing information.
  - Confidentiality: protecting and providing information (2004) – frequently asked questions.
  - Seeking Patients' Consent: the ethical considerations.
  - Serious Communicable Diseases.
  - Withholding and Withdrawing Life-prolonging Treatments: good practice in decision-making.
  - Research: the role and responsibilities of doctors.
  - Making and Using Visual and Audio Recordings of Patients.
  - Advertising.

2   BMA/Law Society (2004) *Assessment of Mental Capacity: guidance for doctors and lawyers* (2e). BMA, London.

3   Royal Society for Mentally Handicapped Children and Adults (1989) *Competency and Consent to Medical Treatment: report of the Working Party.* Royal Society for Mentally Handicapped Children and Adults, London.

4   Department of Health (2001) *Reference Guide to Consent for Examination or Treatment.* Department of Health, London.

5   Medical Protection Society (2002) *Consent: a comprehensive guide for juniors.* Medical Protection Society, London and Leeds.

6   Federation of Royal Colleges of Physicians of the UK (2004) *Good Medical Practice for Physicians.* Federation of Royal Colleges of Physicians of the UK, London.

7   Royal College of Surgeons of England (2000) *Good Surgical Practice.* Royal College of Surgeons of England, London.

8   Senate of Surgery of Great Britain and Ireland (1997) *The Surgeon's Duty of Care.* Senate of Surgery of Great Britain and Ireland, London.

Chapter 5

Financial decisions

Power of attorney

A competent person can authorise someone else to make decisions about his/her financial affairs including property, shares, money, etc. (a proxy decision maker). The person who is handing over power is known as a *donor*, the person who is thus appointed as a legal representative is known as the *donee* or *attorney* and the legal process of transferring power is known as *power of attorney*. Anyone can be a donor providing that they are 18 or over and are mentally capable. An attorney must be 18 or over, of sound mind and not bankrupt at the time the attorney signs the document.

Power of attorney is a legal document and is of two types: ordinary power of attorney and enduring power of attorney.[1-3]

Ordinary power of attorney (OPA)

OPA authorises one or more people to handle your financial affairs so long as you are able to supervise their actions or you need someone to act on your behalf for a temporary period, e.g. you are on holiday or physically ill. This may be a general power without restriction or it may only give limited power to do a specific act, e.g. to sell a house. However, whether the OPA is a general one or is limited, it is only valid while you are capable of giving instructions. It will end if:

- you revoke the power
- you become mentally incapacitated and no longer able personally to supervise or direct the attorney
- the power is time limited and the time has expired
- the power is limited to a specific task, which has been completed
- the attorney(s) themselves die or become incapacitated.

Enduring power of attorney (EPA)

EPA is a similar legal document, but the only difference from OPA is that it will continue even if the person no longer has the mental capacity, provided that it is registered with the Public Guardianship Office (PGO). The donor can decide whether the attorney will start working now and continue after he/she has become mentally incapable in the future or only if he/she becomes mentally incapable some time in the future.

As with the OPA, EPA must be signed (by both donor and attorney) while the donor is capable of understanding the nature and effect of creating an enduring power – otherwise the power will not be valid.

Like OPA, EPA can be general or limited and to ensure greater security, it is advisable to restrict the use of the EPA until after it has been registered with the PGO, which has the administrative functions for the financial affairs of people who lack the capacity to manage their own finances.

As soon as the attorney(s) has reason to believe that the donor is, or is becoming, mentally incapable, he/she (or they) should apply to the PGO to have the EPA registered and prior to that the attorney(s) must send the notice of *intention to register* to the donor and at least three of the donor's nearest relatives.

The donor can revoke an EPA at any time provided he/she has mental capacity. However, an EPA cannot be cancelled or revoked without the court's consent once it has been registered.

The EPA will remain valid until one of the following events occurs:

- the death of either the donor or the sole attorney
- the bankruptcy of the attorney
- revocation before registration by the donor or by the PGO after registration
- disclaimer by the attorney
- mental incapacity of the attorney.

If an adult becomes *mentally incompetent* to manage his/her financial affairs any more and has not granted an EPA then an application for *receivership* may need to be made to the *Court of Protection* for legal handling of financial affairs on his/her behalf.

The current registration fee for EPA is £220 made payable to the PGO. However, if the assets (i.e. bank accounts and shares) are less than £16 000 and there is no property, the PGO would normally reduce some of the registration fee. Anyone with assets of less than £12 250 should have their fee remitted in full and in the case of capital between £12 250 and £16 000 the fee can be reduced to £70.

Court of Protection (CP)

The CP is an office of the *Supreme Court* (not the High Court) and its function is to protect the property and financial affairs of people who are by reason of mental disorder incapable of dealing with their own affairs. The CP is staffed by judges and officers who are experienced in dealing with matters concerning property, and nominated by the Lord Chancellor. The CP's jurisdiction extends to England and Wales. Separate arrangements exist for Scotland and Northern Ireland. It is not normally necessary to appear before the CP as its business is usually conducted by post. The CP functions through its administrative arm, the Public Guardianship Office (PGO).[1-3]

Public Guardianship Office (PGO)

The PGO is the administrative arm of the Court of Protection and part of the Department of Constitutional Affairs. It is also responsible for the registration of EPA.

The CP and PGO would only become involved if something needed to be done either to protect the client's (patient's) assets or to enable them to be used for the benefit of the client. The CP/PGO has the general function to 'do or secure to do all such things as appear necessary and expedient':

- for the maintenance and other benefit of the patient
- for the maintenance or other benefit of members of the patient's family
- for making provisions for other persons or purposes to whom, or which, the patient might be expected to provide if he were not mentally disordered or
- otherwise for administering the patient's affairs.

The court has control over all the property and affairs of a patient under its jurisdiction and it must be consulted when any decision has to be taken in relation to the patient's property or finances. The court may appoint a receiver. In case of small assets (< £16 000) it may make a *short order* regarding the patient's affairs, in place of a *receivership order*. However, these are discretionary and will only be considered after the court has received the application.

The effect of involvement of the CP and PGO in the management and administration of the financial affairs of a person suffering from mental incapacity is to give proper legal authority to the person whom the court appoints as *receiver* to deal fully with the patient's financial affairs. A *receiver*, in law, is defined as a person appointed by a court to manage property – pending the outcome of litigation, during infancy of the owner, or after the owner has been declared bankrupt or of unsound mind.

In the majority of cases the CP is only involved on the appointment of the receiver. However, the PGO will assess the patient's needs and notify the patient about the application for receivership before the CP appoints a receiver and all subsequent directions regarding the administration of the patient's estate are given by the PGO as an administrative rather than judicial act.

The current cost includes a commencement fee (to be sent along with the application form) of £230 and a receivership appointment fee (payable when the court appoints the receiver for the first time) of £300. (In the case of a short order you only need to pay the commencement fee of £70.) There is also an annual administration fee payable to the PGO of £230.

Receivership

Receivership is the function of a receiver. The application to the court for receivership is normally made by the patient's nearest relative or a friend, but an application may be made by others such as a solicitor, accountant, bank manager or local authority. In the case of a large or costly property it is advisable to make the application through a solicitor. Once appointed the receiver takes control of the patient's affairs and property and acts on the patient's behalf in accordance with the court's instructions.

The *role* of a receiver is as follows:

- responsible for collecting the patient's income and paying bills
- should administer the patient's affairs in the best interests of the patient
- should try to be aware of the patient's needs and wishes
- should use the patient's money for the patient's benefit (in the widest sense) during the patient's lifetime

- should consult with the patient, as far as is reasonable and practicable, about how the patient would like his/her money spent
- accountable to the PGO, usually on an annual basis, for their financial dealings with the patient's money.

The following are the *limitations* of power of a receiver:

- cannot deal with transactions involving capital assets, legal proceedings, making loans or gifts without prior approval from the PGO
- does not have power over the 'person' of the patient and cannot authorise an operation, medical treatment, or where the patient should live
- cannot stop a patient getting married or making a will, although the receiver should notify the PGO about these happenings
- the powers of a receiver cease on the death of the patient.[1-3]

References

1   Department of Health and Welsh Office (1999) *Mental Health Act 1983: Code of Practice.* Department of Health and Welsh Office, London.
2   Jones RM (2004) *Mental Health Act Manual* (9e). Sweet and Maxwell, London.
3   Age Concern England website: www.ageconcern.org.uk.

Chapter 6

Compulsory detention and treatment

Compulsory powers in the community (guardianship)

Guardianship is the functions and powers of a guardian. From a *legal point*, a guardian is defined as a person legally appointed to manage the affairs of a person incapable of acting for himself, as a minor or person of unsound mind.

Under the Mental Health Act 1983, from a *social welfare point*, a guardian is a local authority or a person accepted by it as having the powers to require a mentally disordered person to live at a specified place, attend for treatment and be accessible to a doctor or social worker.

The guardianship powers in this Act are largely based on recommendations made by the Royal Commission. The Commission argued that 'care outside hospital should usually be on the basis of persuasion to accept help and advice and take advantage of arrangements for employment and training', and recommended 'where a person's unwillingness to receive training or social help could not be overcome by persuasion it would be appropriate to place him under guardianship'.[1]

Guardianship powers are needed for a number of mentally disordered people who do not require treatment in hospital but need close supervision and some control in the community, including people who neglect themselves to the point of seriously endangering their health.

The purpose of guardianship is to enable patients to receive care in the community where it cannot be provided without the use of compulsory powers. It provides a framework, as part of the overall care and treatment plan, for working with a patient to achieve as independent a life as possible.

Guardianship is *not* a child-centred jurisdiction. It applies to patients who are *at least 16 years old* (predominantly those over 65 years of age) and who are suffering from mental illness, psychopathic disorder, severe mental impairment or mental disorder of a nature or degree which warrants reception into guardianship, and where it is also necessary in the interests of the welfare of the patient or for the protection of others.

Guardianship *applications (section 7)*: section 7 of the Mental Health Act 1983 provides for guardianship under the auspices of a local social services authority (or a named individual accepted by the local social services authority) on the recommendation of two doctors and an application by an approved social worker or nearest relative. The application must be made within 14 days after getting the second medical opinion. Under section 37 a court can also make a guardianship order. In 99% of cases in England, the guardian is a local authority. One very important point to note is that *the PGO has nothing to do with this guardianship*.

The *powers* of a guardian *(section 8)* are:

- the power to require the patient to reside at a specified place
- the power to require the patient to attend specified places for medical treatment, occupation, education or training
- the power to require access to be given to the patient by a doctor, approved social worker or other specified person.

A patient may be kept under guardianship for an initial period of six months and this may be renewed for a further period of six months, then for yearly periods.

A patient shall cease to be subject to guardianship, if an order for his discharge is made by his responsible medical officer, by the responsible local social services authority or by his nearest relative.

Detained patients and patients who are subject to guardianship may be transferred between hospitals and guardians or between detention in hospital and guardianship.

A person who has lost mental capacity as a result of a physical illness (e.g. a stroke) but is not mentally disordered cannot be a subject of guardianship. Similarly, it is not possible for a person with a learning disability whose mental impairment is not associated with abnormally aggressive or seriously irresponsible conduct to be placed under guardianship.

Consideration should be given to making an application for receivership to the Court of Protection for patients who are incapable, by reason of mental disorder, of managing their financial affairs.

Part IV of the Mental Health Act 1983 sets out circumstances in which patients detained under the Act be treated without consent for their mental disorder, but it has no application to treatment for physical disorders unrelated to the medical disorder, which remains subject to the common-law principles.

It is possible for persons who are not necessarily mentally disordered to be compulsorily admitted to a hospital or a residential care facility under the provisions of section 47 of the National Assistance Act 1948. The local authority (district council or county council/borough) can only make an application under section 47 if the community physician has certified to the authority that he is satisfied after 'thorough enquiry and consideration' that it is necessary to remove the person from his/her premises on the following grounds:

- that the person is suffering from grave chronic disease or, being aged, infirm or physically incapacitated, is living in insanitary conditions *and*
- that the person is unable to devote to himself, and is not receiving from other persons, proper care and attention *and*
- that his removal from home is necessary, either in his own interests or for preventing injury to health of, or serious nuisance to, other persons.

If the court finds that the grounds are satisfied, then it may order giving authority for the person's 'detention and maintenance' in a suitable hospital or care home for an initial period up to three months with the court having the power to extend it for a further three months.

However, neither this 1948 Act nor the common law provides authority for medical treatment to be given to a mentally capable person who has been removed from his home under section 47, without his/her consent.[1,2]

Under the proposal of the *Mental Health Bill 2004*, guardianship would be abolished and the automatic link between compulsory treatment and detention in hospital would be broken, allowing patients to be treated in the setting most appropriate to them.

Compulsory admission to hospital

Under the *Mental Health Act 1983*, certain mentally disordered patients can be compulsorily detained in hospital for the purpose of assessment and necessary treatment.[1-3]

Part II of the Act

This provides for compulsory detention of patients for necessary assessment and treatment planning. The relevant sections are 2, 3, 4, 5(2), 5(4) and 136(2). The approved social workers (ASWs) of the patient play the central role. An ASW has the overall responsibility for coordinating the process of assessment of a patient and he/she is the most suitable person to make an application for admission of the patient. However, it is a statutory requirement that the ASW should consult with the nearest relatives of the patient, unless it is not reasonably practicable. An application for admission for assessment must be based on the written recommendations of two medical practitioners who testify that the patient is suffering from mental disorder of a nature warranting his detention in hospital, at least for a limited period, and ought to be so detained in the interests of his own health or safety or to protect others.

Section 2 (admission for assessment) authorises the patient's detention for assessment up to a maximum of 28 days. The criteria for section 2 are as follows:

- The diagnosis and prognosis of patient's condition is unclear.
- There is a need to carry out an inpatient assessment in order to formulate a treatment plan.
- A judgement is needed as to whether the patient will accept treatment on a voluntary basis after admission.
- A judgement has to be made as to whether a particular treatment proposal, which can only be administered to the patient under Part IV of the Act, is likely to be effective.

Section 3 (admission for treatment) authorises the detention of the patient beyond the 28-day period for treatment and after-care under supervision will only be available if the patient is admitted under section 3. The criteria for section 3 are:

- the patient is suffering from mental illness, severe mental impairment, psychopathic disorder or mental impairment of a nature or degree which makes it appropriate for him to receive medical treatment in hospital *and*
- in the case of psychopathic disorder or mental impairment that such treatment is likely to alleviate or prevent a deterioration of his condition *and*
- that it is necessary for the health or safety of other persons that he should receive such treatment, and that it cannot be provided unless he is detained under this section.

Section 4 makes provision for admission for assessment in a genuine emergency, where there is not enough time to get a second medical recommendation. However, an appropriate second medical opinion must be sought as soon as practicable after admission of the patient.

Section 5(2) allows doctors to hold power and authorise the detention of a patient in the hospital for up to *72 hours*. The section cannot be used for an outpatient attending a hospital's A&E department. Usually this power cannot be renewed. Section 5(2) is not an admission section under the Act and it should only be used if at the time it is not possible or safe to use section 2, 3 or 4. When power under section 5(2) is used by a consultant other than a psychiatrist, a psychiatrist must be contacted immediately. Part IV of the Act does not apply to a patient detained under section 5(2).

Section 5(4) empowers a qualified senior nurse (nurse of the *prescribed class*) to lawfully prevent an informal inpatient, receiving medical treatment for mental disorder, from leaving the hospital in a psychiatric emergency where a doctor is not available immediately. This holding power can last up to a maximum of *six hours*, or until a doctor with the power to use section 5(2) arrives, whichever is the earlier, and it cannot be renewed. Part IV of the Act does not apply to patients detained under section 5(4).

Section 136(2) empowers a police officer to remove a patient with psychiatric illness to a place of safety (police station or hospital) to enable the patient to be examined and interviewed by an ASW and for any necessary arrangements for his care and treatment to be made. This power can last up to *72 hours* and subsequent admission to hospital, if necessary, should be under section 2, 3 or 4. Again part IV of the Act does not apply to persons detained under section 136.

Part III of the Act

Part III makes provision for assessment of patients (from prison or a remand centre) concerned with criminal proceedings. The relevant sections are 35, 36, 37, 38, 39, 47 and 48. All professionals involved in the operation of part III of the Act should be aware that psychiatric patients in police or prison custody may be very vulnerable; a prison healthcare centre is not a hospital within the meaning of the Act as comprehensive treatment facilities are rarely available and the provisions of Part IV of the Act do not apply. Assessment for admission of the patient is the responsibility of the doctor but other members involved with the patient's care should be consulted. If the doctor is not sure whether admission to hospital will be beneficial, he/she can recommend an interim hospital order under *section 38* to admit the patient to hospital for up to 12 weeks (extendable up to a maximum of 12 months) for full assessment.

Part IV of the Act

Part IV provides specific statutory authority for forms of medical treatment for mental disorder to be given to most patients liable to be detained, without their consent in certain circumstances. The relevant sections are 57, 58, 62 and 63. The provisions in part IV of the Act are as follows.

- *Section 57 – Treatment requiring the patient's consent and a second opinion:* Any form of psychosurgery such as a lobotomy and surgical implantation of hormones for reduction of male sexual drive will be unlawful unless
  1. the patient consents and
  2. an independent doctor certifies that
     a. the patient is competent to make a decision and
     b. the treatment is likely to benefit the patient. Section 57 applies to all patients and not just those detained in hospital.
- *Section 58 – Treatment requiring the patient's consent or a second opinion:* Any long-term medication (administered longer than three months) and electroconvulsive therapy (ECT) are authorised only if
  1. the patient consents and a doctor certifies that he is competent to do so or
  2. an independent doctor certifies that the patient is incapable of giving consent or has refused to do so but that however '…having regard to the likelihood of the treatment alleviating or preventing a deterioration of his condition, the treatment should be given'. Section 58 applies only to detained patients except those detained under sections 4, 5(2), 5(4), 35, 37(4), 42(2), 73, 74, 135 and 136. Patients detained under these sections can be treated under common law.
- *Section 62 – Urgent treatment:* This makes provisions for urgent treatment of patients mentioned under sections 57 and 58 and violates the usual safeguards under these sections.
- *Section 63 – Treatments that do not require the patient's consent:* However, consent should always be sought. Section 63 authorises psychiatric treatment only, not treatment of any physical illness, which should be treated with the patient's valid consent or under common law. It includes all medical treatments, except for those mentioned under sections 57 and 58, for mental disorder given by or under the direction of the patient's Registered Medical Officer (RMO). This provision applies only to detained patients as under section 58.

Part IV of the Mental Health Act 1983 only applies to patients actually in hospital and there is no provision for continuing care of the patients in the community under this Act. The *Mental Health Act 1995 (Patients in the Community)* grants power to supervise patients returned to the community and, if the patient refuses to comply with his supervised after-care, to return him to hospital.

References

1. Jones RM (2004) *Mental Health Act Manual* (9e). Sweet and Maxwell, London.
2. Department of Health and Welsh Office (1999) *Mental Health Act 1983: Code of Practice.* Department of Health and Welsh Office, London.
3. Brazier M (2003) *Medicine, Patients and the Law* (3e). Penguin Books, Harmondsworth.

Chapter 7

Welfare and healthcare decisions

Introduction

The twentieth century witnessed numerous outstanding discoveries in the fields of medicine and technology, which led to revolutionary advances in the modern practice of medicine. Our understanding of various diseases and their management has improved considerably. Availability of life-support machines, artificial nutrition and hydration, transplants and cardiopulmonary resuscitation has given us the ability to care for very premature infants and to prolong life far beyond what would have been imagined only a few decades ago, and treatments currently only dreamt of will be the norm in this new millennium.

Keeping pace with science and technology, our society is changing with differing social values, expectations and attitudes, which has imposed significant influence on current medical practice. Not so long ago it was rare for patients to be fully informed about a diagnosis of cancer or other life-threatening disease, but that culture and attitude have changed dramatically in recent years. Now patients want to know every detail related to their health and participate in decision making regarding all aspects of their management. Medical paternalism is now replaced by 'the respect for *patients' autonomy*', where *patients have the final say about their treatment*. Keeping pace with time, medical attitudes are also changing.

Until very recently, the medical profession stood very high in public esteem and the popularity polls of professionals regularly resulted in doctors at the top of the poll. The last two decades of the twentieth century dealt a body blow to the medical profession in the United Kingdom. Scandal after scandal (e.g. the Bristol baby heart scandal, the Alder Hey organ retention scandal, the striking off the medical register of a rude gynaecologist after years of gross malpractice, the conviction of the GP Harold Shipman, the conviction of the nurse Beverley Allitt, etc.) beset doctors and nurses and health professionals felt under siege. Doctors, once accorded a godlike status, are often reviled in the media as pariahs.[1]

For so long, doctors' professional conduct was regulated by professional self-regulation principles set by a 'responsible body' and any medical negligence case against a doctor was judged by a test called the *Bolam test* ('A doctor would not be considered negligent if their practice conformed to that of a responsible body of medical opinion held by practitioners skilled in the field in question'). However, in several recent cases this professional self-regulation has been questioned and the 'responsible body of medical opinion' has been criticised. The tradition of self-regulation by the profession alone has been eroded and it is now clear that *the court will be the final arbiter of what constitutes responsible practice*, although the standards set by the health professions for their members will still be influential.[2]

As in any other field, medical advancement has brought some inherent disadvantages with it. Because of the availability of various sophisticated treatment options, doctors and at times patients are confused by the dilemma as to which option to use or not. This has led to a fear among patients of overtreatment at the end of life, mistrust in medical technology or lack of confidence that health professionals will recognise when enough is enough. This acted as a stimulus for patients for making end-of-life decisions in accordance with patients' autonomy to decide what will happen to their own body. End-of-life decisions may be a *living will* or *voluntary euthanasia* (assisted dying).

Living wills

A *living will* is a document, made voluntarily by a competent individual over 18, in which he/she stipulates which treatments he or she would like to receive or refuse in a given set of circumstances in the future when they are no longer able to make decisions or communicate their preferences.

The Lord Chancellor (1997) described a living will as 'a health care decision intended to have effect when a patient loses capacity'.[3]

The Law Commission (1995) used the term *advance statements* because it did not wish to suggest that these anticipatory decisions must always be made in writing.

When 'living wills' was first introduced to the UK, by the Voluntary Euthanasia Society in the early 1980s, they were called *advance directives* because this concept was readily understood by doctors.

The British Medical Association first issued guidelines in 1992 and in 1995 amended and defined advance statements as 'a mechanism whereby competent people give instructions about what is to be done if they subsequently lose the capacity to decide or to communicate'.[3]

Where these advance statements are limited to identifying the treatments a patient would not be willing to accept, the term *advance refusal* is most appropriately used.

The term 'living will' was first coined by Louis Kutner at a meeting of the Euthanasia Society of America in 1967. Livings wills evolved in the USA, where the first statute was the California Natural Death Act 1976.

Living wills cannot demand treatment that would not be appropriate or is illegal. They also cannot refuse 'basic care' such as washing, cleaning and keeping warm, the offer of pain relief and the offer of being fed. At present there is no statute in the UK governing living wills, but they are recognised in common law.

A person can cancel or change his/her living will at any time provided he/she is still competent to make an informed decision.

Criteria for a *valid living will* are as follows:

• The person must be over 18 and mentally competent while making the will.
• The person must be fully informed about the nature and consequences of the will before making it.
• The person made it clear that the living will should apply to all situations or circumstances that may arise in future.
• The person was not pressurised or influenced by anyone else when he/she made the living will.

- The living will has not been changed, either verbally or in writing.
- The person is now incapable of making any decision because he/she is unconscious or otherwise unfit.

The ethical debate surrounding living wills focuses on whether or not suicide is a reasonable choice for an individual to make. Although living wills were initially linked with the euthanasia movement, it is important to recognise that they are separate issues. The underlying philosophy of a living will is *neither the right to die nor the right to live, but the right to choose for oneself*. This is one of the most important components of patients' autonomy. While respecting patients' autonomy is vitally important, it is also true that healthcare professionals always have a duty to act for the patient's best interests, integral to which are preserving life, restoring health and minimising suffering.

While doctors are not bound by a living will to provide a particular treatment (which might be inappropriate), case law is now clear that an *advance refusal of treatment*, which is valid and applicable to subsequent circumstances in which the patient lacks capacity, is *legally binding*. If there is any doubt about the validity of an advance refusal a ruling should be sought from the court.[1,3]

Voluntary euthanasia (assisted dying/physician-assisted suicide)

Euthanasia (*eu* = easy + *thanatos* = death), popularly known as mercy killing, is defined as 'the act of killing someone painlessly, especially to relieve suffering from an incurable illness'.

At the same time, deliberately taking the life of another person, irrespective of whether that person is dying or not, constitutes the crime of *murder*. Accordingly, as per current English law, any doctor who, no matter how compassionately, practises voluntary euthanasia or assists a suicide can be charged with murder, which could expose the doctor to a term of imprisonment of 14 years. However, currently euthanasia is a legal practice in some countries like the Netherlands, Belgium, Switzerland and the Oregon state of the USA.

Euthanasia can be either *active* or *passive* and both of these can be of three types – *voluntary*, *non-voluntary* and *involuntary*.

- *Active euthanasia* – involves a deliberate act (*an act of commission*) designed to shorten life, by however short a span.
- *Passive euthanasia* – is *an act of omission* where life (and suffering) of a dying person is shortened by withholding life-support treatment.
- *Voluntary euthanasia* – where the act of killing is done at the patient's own considered and persistent request.
- *Non-voluntary euthanasia* – refers to ending the life of someone unable to express his/her own view on prolongation of life at the relevant time and a proxy makes a decision on his/her behalf.
- *Involuntary euthanasia* – involves the act of killing a person without his/her or proxy authority.

The *Assisted Dying of the Terminally Ill Bill 2004* was introduced by internationally respected human rights lawyer Lord Joffe and it is currently being considered by a Select Committee of the House of Lords. This Bill, if enacted, would legalise assisted dying in the UK. It will 'enable a competent adult who is suffering unbearably as a result of a terminal illness to receive medical assistance to die at his own considered and persistent request; and to make provision for a person suffering from a terminal illness to receive pain relief medication'. It will be the responsibility of the 'attending physician' (*i.e. the physician who has the primary responsibility for the care of the patient and treatment of the patient's illness*), at the patient's request, either to provide the patient with the means to end the patient's life or, if the patient is unable to do so, to end the patient's life.

The *important points* to consider here are:

- the accuracy of the diagnosis of the, often very complex, reasons for the request for assisted dying
- the patient is competent to make an informed decision based upon an accurate understanding of the situation
- any possibility that the request for hastening death may be in response to real or perceived, explicit or implicit, external pressures, which may be internalised as the desire not to be a burden to others
- the practicalities of assisted dying, including training of necessary staff and subsequent audits.

There is an ongoing national debate on this topical issue and the arguments for and against the Bill are as follows.

Arguments for the Bill:

- There is a clinical need for assisted dying. Several surveys in the last decade revealed that the practice of covert euthanasia is common in the UK and about 12% of doctors admitted involvement in this practice.
- There is a need to change the law to legalise the practice of covert euthanasia and make it open, so that it could be assessed and audited. According to current English law, assisting a suicide is a criminal offence leading to life imprisonment.
- It supports the key principle of modern medical practice, i.e. patients' autonomy.
- Concerns regarding potential adverse effects of the Bill (changing social attitude towards vulnerable people like the elderly, the handicapped and the mortally ill; misdiagnosis of depression and other treatable conditions as terminal illness; imposing undue external pressure on terminally ill people; lack of initiative to improve palliative care services; undermining the doctor–patient relationship of trust; widespread fraud and abuse of the legislation and devaluing the doctrine of sanctity of life) have not been evident from the experiences in the countries where assisted dying is legally practised.

Arguments against the Bill:

- There is no need for such a Bill, which proposes to legalise certain categories of killing. It is suggested that the Bill will bring the covert practice of euthanasia into the open; but it was not reflected by the 2001 survey from the Netherlands where about half of the cases of euthanasia and assisted suicide went unreported. End-of-life issues raise questions of value at the most basic level. We need a better social support system, a better palliative care set-up and a system of proper assessment of the terminally ill whose suffering is usually multifactorial.

- The Bill is morally unjustifiable. There is a real concern about the vulnerable group being less worthy of living and seeing themselves as such. If the moral case for euthanasia rests on the autonomy of terminally ill patients, it will be an injustice if patients with non-terminal illnesses, who consider their lives no longer worth living, are not allowed to have the benefit of death.
- We are born dependent on others and we die dependent on others. As a social creature, autonomy must be exercised in the context of social obligations. One's life is one's own is not an argument that one has the moral right to choose to end it. Euthanasia should not be just another consumer product to demand from the supermarket of life.
- There is a real concern about the undermining effect of the Bill on the doctor–patient relationship at a time when doctors in the UK are already under intense media criticism.

Conclusion: We definitely need better palliative care facilities and social supports. Suicidal people should not be confirmed in their own estimate of their lives' value; instead they should be supported and protected, whatever their physical condition. However, it is also true that universal availability of excellent palliative care services can never eliminate all such rational and persistent requests for euthanasia and maintenance of legal prohibition on this practice exacts a high price on some individuals and unacceptably violates their autonomy.[1,4]

References

1   Brazier M (2003) *Medicine, Patients and the Law* (3e). Penguin Books, Harmondsworth.
2   Department of Health (2001) *Reference Guide to Consent for Examination or Treatment.* Department of Health, London.
3   Wilson L (1999) Living wills. *Nursing Times Monographs.* **7.**
4   Tallis R and Saunders J (2004) The Assisted Dying for the Terminally Ill Bill 2004. *Clinical Medicine.* November/December. **4** (6): 534–40.

Chapter 8

Mental Capacity Bill 2004

The *Mental Capacity Bill*, introduced to Parliament on 17 June 2004 by the Department for Constitutional Affairs, creates a new legal framework for decision making to protect adults who lack mental capacity and those caring for them.

The Bill outlines the following *principles*:

- *A presumption of capacity* – every adult has the right to make his/her own decisions and must be assumed to have capacity to do so unless proved otherwise.
- *An individual's right to be supported to make their own decisions* – people must be given all appropriate help before concluding that they are incapable of making their own decision. This may include involvement of people close to the patient, specialist colleagues like speech and language therapists or learning disability teams, and independent advocates or supporters.
- *An individual's right to make what might be seen as eccentric or unwise decisions* – a competent adult must retain the right to make what might be seen as eccentric or unwise decisions, even those which may lead to their death.
- *Best interests* – anything done for or on behalf of people without capacity must be done in their best interests.
- *Least restrictive interventions* – anything done for or on behalf of people without capacity should be the least restrictive of their basic rights and freedoms.

An important change that the new mental capacity legislation will bring in is that, just as an adult is able to choose someone to take *financial decisions* on his/her behalf, he/she will also be able to choose someone to take *welfare and healthcare decisions* on his/her behalf.

The Bill *enshrines in law the current best practice* and it *will provide legal basis* in the following ways:

- *Best interests* – incapacitated people's best interests are key to the whole Bill. In order to be in the patient's best interests the treatment must be:
  - necessary to save life or to prevent a deterioration or ensure an improvement in the patient's physical or mental health and
  - in accordance with a practice accepted at the time by a responsible body of medical opinion skilled in the particular form of treatment in question. The Bill will also provide a checklist of factors that decision makers must work through in deciding a person's best interests. The best interests checklist is as follows:
  - likely future capacity
  - past and present wishes and feelings of patient
  - need to permit and encourage patient to participate or improve ability to do so
  - views of other people close to patient as to patient's past and present feelings

– least restrictive way of achieving purpose of intervention.

- *General authority* – this provides the legal basis for a person to act on behalf of an adult who lacks capacity. The Bill will clarify that a person acting under the 'general authority' does not have a new authority to intervene in the life of someone who lacks capacity, but that this protects carers from liability when they act in the best interests of a person who cannot consent. The 'general authority' will be renamed, as there have been concerns about how this might be interpreted.
- *Lasting power of attorney (LPA)* – LPA will be established, allowing people to appoint an attorney to act on their behalf if they should lose capacity in the future. A person can choose to apply the LPA to welfare, healthcare and financial matters.
- *Court-appointed deputies* – the Bill will create a system of court-appointed deputies to replace and extend the current system of receivership in the Court of Protection. Deputies will be able to take decisions on welfare, healthcare and financial matters as determined by the court.
- *Advance decisions* – this will confirm the legal basis for people to make a decision to refuse treatment if they should lose capacity in the future. The Bill sets out the circumstances in which advance decisions may be followed by doctors, together with safeguards that will seek to ensure that the person making the advance decision was fully informed and that it has not changed over time.
- *Criminal offence* – the Bill introduces a new criminal offence of neglect or ill treatment that can be used against anyone who has ill-treated or wilfully neglected a person who lacks capacity. A person found guilty of such an offence may be liable to a term up to two years' imprisonment.
- *New Court of Protection* – the Bill will establish a new court with jurisdiction to consider applications for financial decisions and serious healthcare issues (such as sterilisation for contraception), which are currently dealt with by the High Court. The practical working of the court will be designed around the needs of the person lacking capacity.
- *New Public Guardian* – the Public Guardian will be the registering authority for LPA and deputies. He/she will supervise deputies appointed by the court, and provide information to help the court make decisions. He/she will register LPA and, working together with other agencies such as police and social services, will respond to any concerns raised about the way in which the LPA is being operated by the donee.

The Bill will *not* change the law:

- on euthanasia – this is, in any case, not a legal concept: it will remain unlawful to take a person's life, in all the same circumstances as now; the Bill will make this explicit
- on withdrawal of artificial nutrition and hydration from someone in a permanent vegetative state
- in relation to detention under the Mental Health Act.[1]

Reference

1   Mental Capacity Bill 2004. The United Kingdom Parliament (House of Commons) website: www.publications.parliament.uk.

Chapter 9

Medical standards of fitness to drive

Introduction

There are many medical conditions which are likely to cause sudden disabling events at the wheel or inability to safely control the vehicle. In the interest of road safety those who suffer from any of these conditions should not drive. In the United Kingdom, the *Driver and Vehicle Licensing Agency (DVLA)* has produced detailed guidance on these issues and it is updated every six months. It is the duty of the licence holder or the applicant to notify the DVLA of any such medical condition, which may affect safe driving. However, as doctors we should be able to advise our patients about whether or not their medical condition is notifiable to the DVLA, and also the expected outcome of medical enquiries. I am going to discuss in brief the very basics of this issue and their implications for only a few very common medical conditions we manage in our day-to-day practice. For detailed and up to date information, the reader is referred to the DVLA website: www.dvla.gov.uk.

Background

The legal basis of fitness to drive lies in the *Road Traffic Act 1988* and the *Motor Vehicles (Driving Licences) Regulations 1996*. The types of disabilities, categories of vehicles and groups of licence holders have been clarified by the DVLA as follows.

Types of disabilities

- *Prescribed disability* – is one that is a legal bar to the holding of a licence, unless certain conditions are met (e.g. epilepsy).
- *Relevant disability* – is any medical condition that is likely to render the person a source of danger while driving (e.g. visual field defect).
- *Prospective disability* – is any medical condition which, because of its progressive or intermittent nature, may cause the driver to have a prescribed or relevant disability in the course of time (e.g. insulin-treated diabetes).

A driver with a prospective disability may only hold a driving licence subject to medical review in one, two or three years depending upon the circumstances. Drivers with physical disabilities require appropriate adaptations for safe driving and these adaptations are now coded and entered on the licence.

Categories of vehicles

- *Category A* – motorcycles.

- *Category B* – cars.
- *Category C* – lorries.
- *Category D* – buses.
- *Category E* – a trailer, attached to either category B, C or D.

(Some other categories: *F* = agricultural tractors, *G* = road rollers, *H* = mowing machine or vehicle controlled by a pedestrian, *L* = electric vehicles, *N* = vehicles used for very short distances on public roads and *P* = mopeds.)

Groups of drivers (licence holders)

- *Group 1* – includes drivers having licences for category A and B vehicles.
- *Group 2* – includes drivers having licences for category C and D vehicles.

Group 1 licences are normally issued from age 17 to age 70, until restricted to a shorter duration on medical reasons. There is no upper age limit but, after age 70, renewal is necessary every three years.

Group 2 licences are normally issued from age 21 and valid until age 45. They are renewable every five years to age 65 and thereafter renewable annually.

The DVLA does not issue licences for taxis, ambulances or emergency service vehicles. The Medical Commission on Accident Prevention recommends group 2 licences for these categories as an occupational health policy.[1]

GMC guidelines

Legally, it is the responsibility of the licence holder or the applicant to notify the DVLA of any medical condition which may affect safe driving. However, in some circumstances the licence holder cannot or may not do this. Under these circumstances the GMC has issued clear guidelines as follows:

1 The DVLA is legally responsible for deciding if a person is medically unfit to drive. They need to know when driving licence holders have a condition which may, now or in the future, affect their safety as a driver.
2 Therefore, where patients have such conditions, you should:
   - Make sure that the patients understand that the condition may impair their ability to drive. If a patient is incapable of understanding this advice, for example because of dementia, you should inform the DVLA immediately.
   - Explain to patients that they have a legal duty to inform the DVLA about the condition.
3 If patients refuse to accept the diagnosis or the effect of the condition on their ability to drive, you can suggest that they seek a second opinion, and make appropriate arrangements for them to do so. You should advise patients not to drive until the second opinion has been obtained.
4 If patients continue to drive when they are not fit to do so, you should make every reasonable effort to persuade them to stop. This may include telling their next of kin.
5 If you do not manage to persuade patients to stop driving, or you are given or find evidence that a patient is continuing to drive contrary to advice, you

should disclose relevant medical information immediately, in confidence, to the medical adviser at the DVLA.

6   Before giving information to the DVLA you should inform the patient of your decision to do so. Once the DVLA has been informed, you should also write to the patient, to confirm that a disclosure has been made.[2]

DVLA regulations

The licence holder or the applicant must notify the DVLA, or the responsible doctor should do that according to the above GMC guidelines. The final decision is to be taken by the DVLA after necessary assessment and investigations. Some examples of DVLA regulations on driving in a few common medical disorders are given in Table 9.1. For further detailed and up-to-date information the reader is again referred to the DVLA website as above.[1]

Table 9.1 DVLA regulations on driving

Disorders	Group 1 licence	Group 2 licence
Loss of consciousness (LOC) due to simple faint /syncope (presence of typical provocation, prodrome and postural nature)	No driving restriction	No driving restriction
LOC likely to be unexplained syncope and low risk of recurrence (normal cardiac and neurological examinations and ECG)	Driving permitted four weeks after the event	Driving permitted three months after the event
LOC likely to be unexplained syncope and high risk of recurrence (abnormal findings in cardiac or neurological examination and/or investigations)	Six months off driving if no cause found on detailed cardiac and neurological investigations. Can drive four weeks after the event if the cause has been identified and treated	Licence revoked for one year if no cause found on detailed cardiac and neurological investigations. Can drive four weeks after the event if the cause has been identified and treated
Unwitnessed (presumed) LOC with seizure markers (LOC > 5 mins, amnesia > 5 mins, tongue biting, incontinence, injury, post-ictal confusion or headache, etc.)	One year refusal or revocation	Five years' refusal or revocation
LOC with no clinical pointers	Six months refusal or revocation	One year refusal or revocation
Epilepsy	One year off driving since last seizure	Ten years seizure-free off anti-epileptic drugs, before re-licensing considered

Table 9.1 *continued*

Disorders	Group 1 licence	Group 2 licence
First unprovoked seizure	As above	As above
Provoked seizure from alcohol or illicit drugs	Licence revoked for at least one year from last seizure	Licence revoked for at least ten years from last seizure
Provoked seizure from other causes like reflex anoxia, drug induced, immediately after head injury or within 24 hours of stroke/TIA/ intra-cranial surgery	To be dealt with on an individual basis by the DVLA, depending on the 'liability to epileptic seizures' and successful treatment or removal of the provoking factors	To be dealt with on an individual basis by the DVLA, depending on the 'liability to epileptic seizures' and successful treatment or removal of the provoking factors
Withdrawal of anti-epileptic medications	Advised not to drive from commencement of withdrawal until six months after cessation of treatment	Advised not to drive from commencement of withdrawal until six months after cessation of treatment
Narcolepsy/cataplexy	Cease driving on diagnosis, re-licensing considered after satis-factory control of symptoms	Generally considered unfit for driving permanently
Stroke/TIA	Must not drive for at least one month. No need to notify DVLA, unless there is residual neurological deficit at one month	Notify DVLA. Revocation of licence for at least one year
Chronic neurological disorders (e.g. MS, MND, Parkinson's disease or muscle and movement disorders)	No restriction if regular medical assessment confirms no impairment of driving performance	Revocation if the condition is progressive or disabling, otherwise licensed subject to annual review
Angina (DVLA requirement for a negative ETT – no symptoms or significant ECG changes on com-pletion of three stages in Bruce protocol, off anti-anginal medications for 48 hours. Repeat ETT at least every three years)	Should stop driving if angina at rest or at the wheel. No need to notify DVLA	Continuing symptoms will lead to refusal or revocation of licence. Re-licensing when symptom free and meet the exercise test (ETT) requirement
Myocardial infarction/CABG	Stop driving for at least four weeks. No need to notify DVLA	Disqualified for at least six weeks and re-licensed if meet the above criteria
Cardiac arrhythmias	Stop driving if symptoms likely to cause incapacity. No need to notify DVLA, unless disabling symptoms present	Disqualified until adequate symptoms control for three months and LV ejection fraction > 40%

Table 9.1 *continued*

Disorders	Group 1 licence	Group 2 licence
Permanent pacemaker implantation	Must stop driving for one week	Disqualified from driving for six weeks
Implantable cardioverter defibrillator (ICD) implantation	Licence may be granted under strict criteria and subject to annual review	Disqualified from driving permanently
Insulin-treated diabetes mellitus	Notify DVLA. Licence granted under review for one, two or three years	Disqualified from driving permanently
Alcohol or drug misuse and dependency	Disqualified for at least 6–12 months	Disqualified for at least one to three years
Visual disorders(Legal requirements for safe driving: 1 ability to read a number plate with letters 79.4 mm high at a distance of 20.5 metres (corrected acuity ≥ 6/9) 2 a visual field of at least 120° on horizontal axis and 3 normal binocular vision)	Binocular vision is not a requirement as long as the other requirements are met	Disqualified unless all legal requirements are fulfilled
Profound deafness	No restriction till 70. No need to notify DVLA	Licence is refused or revoked if unable to communicate in an emergency even with the help of a device
Dementia	Must notify DVLA. In early dementia a licence may be issued subject to annual review	Must notify DVLA and the licence will be revoked

CABG: coronary artery bypass graft; ECG: electrocardiogram; ETT: exercise tolerance test; LOC: loss of consciousness; LV: left ventricular; MND: motor neurone disease; MS: multiple sclerosis; TIA: transient ischaemic attack.

References

1 Drivers Medical Unit, DVLA. *At a Glance Guide to the Current Medical Standards of Fitness to Drive.* Drivers Medical Unit, DVLA website: www.dvla.gov.uk.
2 General Medical Council's current documents on 'Duties of a doctor'. Available at www.gmc-uk.org.
   - Good Medical Practice.
   - Confidentiality: protecting and providing information.
   - Confidentiality: protecting and providing information (2004) – frequently asked questions.
   - Seeking Patients' Consent: the ethical considerations.

Chapter 10

Brain death

Introduction

The second half of the twentieth century witnessed one of the most important controversies related to a very fundamental fact of life – *death*. It generated a conceptual crisis on *defining death*, which continued for decades all over the world. 'Modern technology, in its desperate attempts to save life, has produced an entity widely known as *brain death*',[1] which created a conflict with the general public's common philosophical concept of death: 'the irreversible loss of capacity for consciousness and cessation of circulatory and respiratory function'.[1] New terminologies like 'vegetative state', 'whole brain death' and 'brainstem death' evolved. The reader is referred to *ABC of Brain Stem Death* and *The Vegetative State* for detailed accounts on these issues. My intention here is to give a brief overview on 'vegetative state' and 'brainstem death'. However, before that we have to have a clear concept on the following basic facts.[1,2]

Basic concepts

- *Consciousness* is a state of mind encompassing both wakefulness and awareness.
  - *Wakefulness* is a state in which the eyes are open and there is a varying degree of motor arousal, whereas sleep is a state of eye closure and motor quiescence. The centre for wakefulness is situated in the upper brainstem and thalamus.
  - *Awareness* refers to the ability to experience one's own self and the environment. The contents of awareness also include memories, thoughts, emotions and intentions. There is no single clinical sign or laboratory test of awareness. Presence of awareness is deduced from a range of behaviours which indicate that an individual can perceive self and surroundings, frame intentions and communicate. Our understanding of the brain mechanism of awareness is incomplete; however, structures in the cerebral hemispheres clearly play the key role.
- *Coma* is a state of deep unconsciousness in which the eyes are closed and sleep–wake cycles absent. Patients are unrousable, fail to open their eyes spontaneously, express no comprehensible words and neither obey commands nor move their limbs to localise or resist painful stimulation. The *Glasgow Coma Scale (GCS)* score varies from *3 to 8* (E1–2, M1–4, V1–2). Coma is usually transient, lasting hours to days, rarely more than two to four weeks. The common

causes of coma are head injuries, trauma, hypoxia, hypothermia, metabolic or endocrine disturbances, drug or alcohol overdose, intra-cranial infections and brain tumours.

- *Death* – the common philosophical concept of death is 'the irreversible loss of capacity for consciousness and cessation of circulatory and respiratory function'. However, 'irreversible cessation of heartbeat and respiration implies *death of the patient as a whole*. It does not necessarily imply the immediate *death of every cell in the body*'.[1] Similarly, 'irreversible cessation of brainstem function implies *death of the brain as a whole*. It does not necessarily imply the immediate *death of every cell in the brain*'.[1]

Vegetative state

The term *permanent vegetative state (PVS)* was first coined by neurosurgeons Bryan Jennett and Fred Plum in 1972 to describe a condition resulting from severe brain damage. It indicated a state characterised by 'wakefulness without awareness'.

Definition

The *vegetative state (VS)* is characterised by wakefulness with cycles of eye closure and eye opening resembling those of sleep and waking. As a rule, the patient can breathe spontaneously and has a stable circulation. However, close observation does not reveal any sign of awareness or of a functioning mind, i.e. they are unaware of self and environment, cannot communicate with others or form intentions. The state may be a transient stage in the recovery from coma or it may persist until death.

The term *persistent vegetative state* is used when vegetative state continues for four weeks or more.

The common causes of vegetative state are traumatic brain injury, stroke and hypoxic ischaemic brain injury.

The outlook for people in a vegetative state is influenced by their age, underlying cause of the vegetative state and its current duration – the longer the state persists, the lower is the chance of recovery.

At *one month* after traumatic brain injury (e.g. a car crash), people in a vegetative state have a > 50% chance of regaining awareness, whereas those with a non-traumatic cause (e.g. a stroke or cardiac arrest) have a chance of < 20%. Beyond one year following trauma, and beyond six months in non-traumatic cases, the chance of regaining awareness is extremely low.

Patients in the persistent vegetative state should therefore be observed for *12 months after head injury* and *six months after non-traumatic injury* before it is judged to be *permanent vegetative state (PVS)*.

Diagnostic criteria

Preconditions

- Every effort has been made to establish the underlying cause of the condition.

- Possible effects of drugs have been assessed and ruled out.
- Possibility of continuing metabolic disturbances has been considered and excluded.
- Any treatable structural cause (e.g. brain tumour) has been ruled out.
- To diagnose PVS the patient must be assessed by at least two doctors, both of whom are experienced in assessing disorders of consciousness. They should take into account the views of the medical staff, therapists, carers and relatives about the patient's reactions and responses. They should examine the patient separately and record their assessment in the patient's notes.
- The diagnosis of PVS will be confirmed only if there is a unanimous agreement among the medical staff, nursing staff, therapists and the patient's family and friends.
- In case of doubt, the diagnosis of PVS should not be made in a hurry and the patient should be reassessed after an interval. In some cases, an expert clinical neuropsychological assessment should be carried out.

Clinical criteria

- No evidence of awareness of the self or the environment at any time.
- No response of any kind (to visual, auditory, tactile or noxious stimuli) suggesting intention, will or conscious purpose.
- No evidence of understanding or meaningful expression.
- Presence of cycles of eye closure and eye opening giving the appearance of a sleep–wake cycle.
- Preservation of spontaneous respiration and circulation.

Clinical features

- *Compatible features* – cycle of sleep and wakefulness; a range of spontaneous movements including chewing, teeth grinding, swallowing, roving eye movements, purposeless limb movements, smiling, grimacing, making grunting or groaning sounds for no discernible reason and preservation of brainstem reflexes.
- *Compatible but atypical features* – following a moving target for more than a fraction of a second, fixing a target or reacting to visual menace, utterance of a single meaningful word or an epileptic seizure.
- *Incompatible features* – any evidence of a functioning mind like discriminative perception, purposeful action or communicative acts.

Management

Persistent good communication between the medical and nursing staff and the relatives and carers of the patient throughout the course of VS is of utmost importance. The patient's advance refusal of any treatment should be respected and views of those close to the patient are to be considered.

High quality nursing care to avoid the preventable complications of this highly dependent state is the mainstay of management. Standard measures include:

- adequate nutrition and hydration, usually via a feeding tube
- good skin and eye care, oral and dental hygiene

- regular suction to avoid aspiration
- careful management of bowel and bladder incontinence
- passive joint exercises to minimise contractures.

Careful *monitoring and recording of patients' responses* by the staff on a daily basis are essential components of management.

At present, in England and Wales but not in Scotland, prior permission from the court is a legal requirement before *withdrawal of nutrition and hydration* and any life-prolonging treatment is considered. Adequate time should be given to the patient's relatives to understand and consider the implications of such actions.

The normal standards of *palliative care* should be observed to ensure the dignity of death.

Differential diagnosis

The differential diagnosis of a vegetative state includes the conditions shown in Table 10.1.

Brainstem death

Brain death was first described clinically by two French physicians, Mollaret and Goulon, in 1959. The awareness of brain death spread further with the introduction of the Harvard criteria (1968) and subsequently Minnesota criteria (1971). The importance of the brainstem was realised as early as 1964, when Professor Keith Simpson wrote that 'there is life so long as a circulation of oxygenated blood is maintained to live brain stem centers'.[1] Doctors 'were attempting to define and establish beyond reasonable doubt *a state of irreversible damage to the brain stem, the point of no return*'.[1]

The common causes of brainstem death are head injury (50%), intra-cranial (sub-arachnoid and intra-cerebral) haemorrhage (30%), meningitis, encephalitis, brain abscess, brain tumour and judicial hanging. Hypoxia from cardio-respiratory arrest is a rare cause of brainstem death; it usually leads to a vegetative state.

There are *three steps to making a diagnosis of brainstem death*:

- ensuring that certain preconditions have been met
- excluding reversible causes of apnoeic coma and
- confirming brainstem areflexia and persistent apnoea.

Preconditions

Two preconditions have to be met:

- the patient is in apnoeic coma, i.e. unresponsive and on a ventilator
- the cause of coma is irremediable structural brain damage due to a 'disorder which can lead to brain death'.

The *positive diagnosis of coma and its underlying aetiology* is of utmost importance

Table 10.1 Differential diagnosis of vegetative state

Condition	Vegetative state (VS)	Minimally conscious state (MCS)	Locked-in syndrome	Coma	Brainstem death
Awareness	Absent	Present	Present	Absent	Absent
Sleep–wake cycle	Present	Present	Present	Absent	Absent
Response to noxious stimuli	+/−	Present	Present (in eyes only)	+/−	Absent
GCS score	E4, M1–4, V1–2	E4, M1–5, V1–4	E4, M1, V1	E1–2, M1–4, V1–2	E1, M1–3, V1
Motor function	No purposeful movement	Some purposeful verbal or motor behaviour	Volitional vertical eye movements or eyeblink preserved	No purposeful movement	None or only reflex spinal movement
Respiratory function	Typically preserved	Typically preserved	Typically preserved	Variable	Absent
EEG activity	Typically slow-wave activity	Insufficient data	Typically normal	Typically slow-wave activity	Typically absent
Cerebral metabolism (PET)	Severely reduced	Insufficient data	Mildly reduced	Moderate to severely reduced	Severely reduced or absent
Prognosis	Variable: recovery, MCS or death	Variable: recovery, VS or death	Depends on cause, full recovery unlikely	Recovery, VS or death within weeks	Already dead

This table is reprinted from the Report of the Working Party of the Royal College of Physicians (2003), with kind permission from the RCP.[1] EEG = electroencephalography; GCS = Glasgow Coma Scale; PET = positron emission tomography. NB: EEG and PET are not required to make these clinical diagnoses.

and this depends on standard methods of history taking, clinical examination and special investigations.

The nature of brain damage must be *structural*, not functional.

The *irremediable nature of the disorder* is assessed by the extent of structural damage, severity of clinical features and passage of time.

Passage of adequate time between the diagnosis of apnoeic coma and testing for brainstem death is an essential component to establish the irreversible nature of the disorder. This 'minimum adequate time interval' varies from 4 to 100 hours depending on the nature of the underlying disorders. However, the adequate time before testing equals the time it takes to satisfy the preconditions.

Exclusions

The potentially reversible, functional, causes of coma must be excluded:

- therapeutic drug effects (sedatives, hypnotics, muscle relaxants)
- hypothermia (temperature < 35°C)
- metabolic abnormalities
- endocrine abnormalities
- intoxication.

Brainstem death should not be considered in the presence of these conditions. In the case of suspected intoxication it is important to remember the approximate plasma half-lives of the coma-producing drugs and also that the blood concentration may lag significantly behind brain concentration.

Criteria for brainstem death

The following criteria are currently used for testing brainstem death:
- confirmation of absent brainstem reflexes
- confirmation of persistent apnoea
- clinical tests should be performed separately by two experienced practitioners, of whom at least one should be a consultant. In practice these doctors are usually anaesthetists, neurologists, neurosurgeons or intensive care physicians but this is certainly not essential
- neither of the practitioners should be part of the transplant team
- clinical tests should be performed on two separate occasions
- there is no necessary prescribed time interval between the tests.

Clinical tests for absent brainstem reflexes

The following *five brainstem reflexes* must be absent before brainstem death can be diagnosed:

- no papillary response to light
- absent corneal reflex
- no motor response within cranial nerve distribution (no grimacing)
- absent vestibulo-ocular reflex

- absent gag or cough reflex.

Oculo-cephalic reflex (doll's eye phenomenon) is not included in the UK code for testing brainstem death. However, testing for 'dolling' is suggested early in every case. *Presence of dolling is a clear indication of a functioning brainstem* and no further testing is justified.

Oculo-cephalic reflex (doll's eye phenomenon) – this test is contraindicated in suspected cervical spine injury. Standing at the head end of the bed the examiner should hold the patient's head with two hands and gently raise the eyelids with the thumbs. The head is rotated to one side and kept there for 3–4 seconds and then rotated 180° to the opposite side. During the whole procedure, a close watch is kept on what happens to the patient's eyes. In a normal alert person, the eyes will orient with the head within a fraction of a second. In a dead person (brainstem death), the head and eyes will move together. In a person with a normal brainstem but damaged cerebral hemisphere, the test reveals an exaggerated 'release phenomenon'. As the head is rotated, there will be quite obvious deviation of the eyes to the opposite side for 1–2 seconds, followed by a quick realignment of the eyes with the head. This release phenomenon is known as positive doll's eye phenomenon, a clear indication of a functioning brainstem.

Oculo-vestibular reflex (caloric testing) – it requires a wax-free external auditory canal and can be performed in the presence of a perforated tympanic membrane. Irrigation of the tympanic membrane with 20 ml of ice-cold water is recommended. In a dead person (brainstem death), this stimulus should not elicit any eye movement. There will be tonic deviation of the eyes towards the irrigated ear in the presence of a functioning brainstem. Deviation restricted to ipsilateral eye indicates a contralateral internuclear ophthalmoplegia and deviation confined to contralateral eye suggests an ipsilateral sixth cranial nerve palsy. This reflex may be impaired due to end organ (vestibular) damage or CNS (central nervous system) depressant drugs (e.g. sedatives, anticonvulsants, etc.).

Tests for confirmation of persistent apnoea

The ultimate test for brainstem function is the test for apnoea. Apnoea is established by showing that no respiratory movements occur during disconnection from the ventilator, for long enough (= 10 minutes) to ensure that the arterial carbon dioxide tension ($PaCO_2$) rises to a level (> 6.65 kPa or 50 mm Hg) capable of driving any respiratory centre neurones that may still be alive. To ensure this and to prevent hypoxia-induced brain damage during the testing period the following criteria are used:

- preoxygenation with 100% oxygen for 10 minutes
- allow $PaCO_2$ to rise to 5.3 kPa or 40 mm Hg before testing by ventilating for a further five minutes with a mixture of 5% CO_2 and 95% O_2
- disconnect from ventilator
- maintain adequate oxygenation through diffusion oxygenation by delivering oxygen at 6 L/min via an intra-tracheal catheter
- allow $PaCO_2$ to rise above 6.65 kPa
- confirm no spontaneous respiration
- reconnect ventilator.

Once the brainstem death is thus confirmed, cessation of further treatment and final disconnection from the ventilator should be considered after detailed discussion with other healthcare team members and the relatives of the patient.[2]

References

1 Pallis C and Harley DH (1996) *ABC of Brainstem Death* (2e). BMJ Books, London.
2 Royal College of Physicians (2003) *The Vegetative State: guidance on diagnosis and management.* Report of a Working Party of the Royal College of Physicians. Royal College of Physicians, London.

Section 3: Medical ethics and medico-social issues

- Medical ethics
- Medico-social issues

Chapter 11

Medical ethics

Introduction

Ethics is a branch of philosophy that studies *morals, values* and the differences between *right* and *wrong*. Medical ethics is the study of philosophical questions pertaining to the practice of medicine and healthcare. Physicians' medical ethics have long been governed by the *Hippocratic oath*, in which physicians declare that they will not do any harm to their patients. In the modern era the licensing boards and national and international associations hold physicians accountable for their decisions in the practice of medicine.

Changing social values

Since the time of Hippocrates – the Greek physician (460–377 BC) commonly regarded as the *father of medicine* – our society and social values have changed considerably and that has greatly affected our modern practice of medicine and healthcare. Modern medical practice is centred around the key principle of *respect for the autonomy of the patient* – i.e. patients have every right to decide whether or not to undergo any medical intervention even where a refusal may result in harm to themselves or in their own death. Successful relationships between doctors and patients depend on confidence and trust and to establish that trust the doctor must respect patients' autonomy and confidentiality. Medical ethics plays a significant role in all aspects of a successful relationship between doctor and patient.

Common ethical issues

Here are a few *common ethical dilemmas* we face in managing terminally ill patients or seriously ill patients with multiple co-morbidities in our day-to-day clinical practice:

- ample supply of addictive pain-relief medications to terminally ill patients
- attempt at cardio-pulmonary resuscitation (CPR) in the event of arrest
- withholding or withdrawing artificial nutrition and hydration (ANH)
- withholding or withdrawing other life-prolonging treatments including mechanical life-supports for those in permanent vegetative states (PVS).

Some contemporary ethical issues

A few topical issues in medical ethics are:

- assisted dying of the terminally ill (euthanasia)
- potentials of stem-cell research, human cloning and genetic research
- animal experimentation and xeno-transplantations, etc.

Practical guidance

There are no easy ways to get out of these dilemmas. We have to consider a few *important points* to solve these issues rationally.[1,2]

- Good practice guidance is based on doctors' *ethical obligations* to show respect for human life, protect the health of their patients and make their patients' best interests their first concern; at the same time doctors have *legal obligations* to work within the law.
- Doctors should give priority to patients on the basis of their *clinical need* and should follow *non-discrimination* as regards to their age, disability, race, colour, gender, sexuality, culture, beliefs, lifestyle, social or economic status.
- *If the patient has the capacity to make their own decision* – then we are legally bound to respect the patient's autonomy. However, if a patient wishes to have a treatment that, in the doctor's considered view, is not clinically indicated, there is no ethical or legal obligation on the doctor to provide it. The doctor should, however, give the patient a clear explanation of the reasons for his/her view, and respect patients' request to have a second opinion. Similarly, doctors should respect a competent patient's decision to refuse CPR, but they have no obligation to comply with a patient's request to provide CPR if they think that the treatment is futile and burdensome.
- *If the patient does not have the capacity to make their own decision* – in the case of children, persons with parental responsibility can make decisions for them. In case of incompetent adults, the *doctor in charge of the patient's care* should make the decision after consultation with *the healthcare team* and *those close to the patient* (patient's spouse/partner, family and friends, near relative, carer, a person with parental responsibility or a proxy decision maker [Scotland]). However, the following points are to be considered before making a decision in these situations:
  - Patients' *advance statements*/advance directives/living wills.
  - Patients' *best interests* – which are not limited to their 'best medical interests' (severity and prognosis of the illness and associated co-morbidities). Other factors which should be taken into consideration are their wishes and beliefs when competent, their current wishes, general well-being and overall quality of life and cultural and religious beliefs.
  - Views about the patient's preference given by those close to the patient.
  - If there is more than one option (including non-treatment) available, the option which least restricts the patient's future choices while achieving the purpose of intervention should be in the patient's best interest.
- A *second opinion* should be sought where treatment is complex and/or the patient or people close to the patient express doubt about the proposed treatment.
- The final decision about the clinical merits of attempting resuscitation rests with the consultant or general practitioner in charge of the patient's care. However, good consistent communication between the doctor, nurses, patient and

those close to the patient is the key to ensuring that the patient's rights are respected, and misunderstanding and dissent are minimised.

- Confidentiality is central to trust between doctors and patients. Doctors must respect patients' confidentiality and should not disclose private and sensitive information about a patient, whether living or dead, without prior valid consent, unless impracticable or in exceptional circumstances.
- There is a great deal of interplay between medical ethics and medical laws and in many cases there is no distinct boundary between the two. Therefore when there is any doubt, controversy or significant disagreement as regards to proposed treatment, capacity or best interests of the patient, *legal advice* should be sought about applying to the court for a ruling.
- *Statutory regulations* – court approval/ruling is a necessity prior to the following interventions: withdrawal of ANH from a patient in PVS, sterilisation for contraceptive purposes, donation of regenerative tissue such as bone marrow, and where there is doubt as to the patient's capacity or best interests, etc.

References

1   General Medical Council's current documents on 'Duties of a doctor'. Available at www.gmc-uk.org.
    - Good Medical Practice.
    - Confidentiality: protecting and providing information.
    - Confidentiality: protecting and providing information (2004) – frequently asked questions.
    - Seeking Patients' Consent: the ethical considerations.
    - Serious Communicable Diseases.
    - Withholding and Withdrawing Life-prolonging Treatments: good practice in decision-making.
    - Research: the role and responsibilities of doctors.
    - Making and Using Visual and Audio Recordings of Patients.
    - Advertising.
2   Department of Health (2001) *Reference Guide to Consent for Examination or Treatment*. Department of Health, London.

Chapter 12

Medico-social issues

Introduction

Society is becoming more diverse with changing public expectations and health needs. The population is ageing, chronic illness is increasing, prevention becomes more important and a better-informed public wants more control and choice, less waiting, safe and high quality treatment and joined-up services. Technological advances have contributed to better investigation and treatment facilities as well as enabling more care to take place in the home and primary care. Ninety per cent of all patient journeys begin and end in primary care. That is why development of primary care lies at the heart of the NHS Plan.

As a consequence of overall improvement of socio-economic conditions and better medical facilities the life expectancy of the population as a whole has increased considerably and this has led to an expanding elderly population. In addition to their multiple medical problems, they have a number of social problems related to their care, which need multidisciplinary input. Their physical and mental disability related to age and multiple associated medical problems make them incapable of managing even their activities of daily living (ADL), which need help, supervision and care. To fulfil this requirement there has been a parallel development of *social services* along with the *health services*.[1,2] However, social services are not only used by the elderly population; they are shared by younger persons with physical/mental disabilities, serious illnesses and drug and alcohol-related problems. Primary care trusts play the central role in integrating these social and healthcare needs of the people in the community through a dedicated *multidisciplinary workforce* consisting of general practitioners (GPs), specialist nurses, district nurses, general nurses, healthcare assistants, health visitors, physiotherapists, occupational therapists, speech and language therapists, psychologists, dieticians, chiropodists and social workers. This workforce is also helped by community physicians (like psychiatrists, paediatricians, geriatricians, etc.) and various voluntary organisations.

Glossary

Before discussing various available medico-social services in the primary care set-up, I would like to explain a few commonly used terminologies briefly.

Rehabilitation

Rehabilitation is a systematic process of helping a person who has acquired a disability or addiction to restore to normal or near-normal life or to readapt to society or a new job with the help of retraining, therapy or vocational guidance.

The aim is to improve the physical and mental ability of a person to restore maximum possible independence in both their personal and professional life. This is achieved through input from a team of professionals and specialists, known as an integrated multidisciplinary team.

Some examples are: rehabilitating a stroke patient to achieve maximum possible independence in his activities of daily living; helping an alcohol/drug addict with the help of a community alcohol/drug team to readapt to society; or helping a person with a mental illness to readapt to a new job.[3]

Multidisciplinary team (MDT)

Health and social needs are changing mainly due to an increasing elderly population. These elderly patients lie at the centre of a complex mix of interactions between medical, functional, psychological and social needs, which require the input of a multidisciplinary team – *a team of professionals and specialists from different disciplines whose integrated actions make rehabilitation possible.*

A multidisciplinary team is likely to include doctors, nurses, physiotherapists, occupational therapists, speech and language therapists, psychotherapists, dieticians, social workers and some others like specialist nurses, psychiatrists, etc.

All team members meet regularly, usually on a weekly basis, to review the progress of the patients and make realistic targets and decisions on the best way forward. This multidisciplinary team meeting is usually chaired by a geriatrician with his/her knowledge of the medical problems that form the basis of the patient's difficulties and it is often the medical prognosis that influences the team's decisions and the outcome. To run a multidisciplinary meeting successfully, the chairperson must be a good communicator, team leader and a team worker.[3]

Physiotherapy (PT)

Physiotherapy is a form of therapy that uses physical agents like exercise, massage and application of electro-physical modalities to improve the health and well-being of patients. Physiotherapy is a healthcare profession which sees human movement as central to the health and well-being of individuals.

Physiotherapists identify and maximise movement potential through health promotion, preventive healthcare, treatment and rehabilitation. Physiotherapists help and treat people of all ages with physical problems caused by illness, accident or ageing.

Physiotherapists work within hospitals as well as outside the hospital setting – in the community and many other places like industry, special schools, leisure and sports, etc. They work in almost all areas and medical specialities, especially care of the elderly, stroke patients, orthopaedics and intensive care.

Although the core skills of physiotherapists involve manual therapy, therapeutic exercise and application of electro-physical modalities, they have to have an appreciation of psychological, cultural and social factors of their clients, good communication skills and understand the principle of team-working.[4]

Occupational therapy (OT)

Occupational therapy is a form of physical therapy involving the therapeutic use of productive and creative activities (crafts and hobbies) for the treatment and rehabilitation of physically or mentally disabled people.

Occupational therapists work with the disabled, the elderly, newborns, school-aged children, and with anyone who has a permanent or temporary impairment in their physical or mental functioning. The aim of occupational therapy is to help the patient to perform daily tasks in their living and working environments, and to assist them to develop the skills to live independent, satisfying and productive lives.

Occupational therapists, like physiotherapists, work in a variety of settings, both within and outside hospitals.

Interventions used by occupational therapists to achieve greater independence by patients include:

- rehabilitation of neuropsychological deficits, e.g. memory, attention or complex reasoning
- motor function, e.g. weakness or unsteadiness
- sensory function, e.g. vision or perception of touch
- interpersonal skills, e.g. social skills
- environmental manipulation to maximise ability, e.g. to create a suitable home environment for wheelchair users, to make necessary alterations in the home environment for partially sighted patients or patients with visual field defects, to set up an environment containing clues to compensate for memory impairment.

The medium of treatment usually involves the use of *purposeful activities*, which have some meaning and relevance to the patient's lifestyle. These are also known as *occupations* and include routine behaviours associated with work, leisure and self-care.[4]

Speech and language therapy (SLT)

Speech and language therapy is defined as any therapy intended to correct a disorder of speech, especially through the use of exercises and audiovisual aids.

The role of a speech and language therapist (SLT) includes:

- to assess and treat speech, language and communication problems in people of all ages to enable them to communicate to the best of their ability
- to assess and treat people who have eating and swallowing problems
- to work closely with carers, teachers and health professionals including doctors, nurses and psychologists.

SLTs work in a variety of settings – hospital inpatients and outpatients, community health centres, schools, day centres and clients' homes.

SLTs assist children and adults who have any of the following *developmental* (e.g. learning disability, cerebral palsy, cleft palate, etc.) or *acquired* (e.g. stroke, accident, cancer of mouth and throat, dementia, deafness, etc.) speech, language or swallowing problems:

- difficulty producing and using speech
- difficulty understanding and/or using language
- difficulty with feeding, chewing or swallowing
- a stammer
- a voice problem.[4]

Psychology/psychiatry/psychotherapy

There are quite significant differences between psychology, psychiatry and psychotherapy, although there is considerable overlap.

Psychology is the study of people: how they think, how they act, react and interact. Psychology is concerned with the normal functioning of the mind including all aspects of behaviour and thoughts, feelings and motivation underlying such behaviour.

Psychologists deal in the way the mind works and they can specialise in various areas:

- clinical psychology
- counselling psychology
- educational psychology
- forensic psychology
- health psychology
- occupational psychology.

Psychologists are not usually medically qualified and only a small proportion of psychologists directly work with patients.

Psychiatry is the study of mental disorders and their diagnosis, management and prevention. Psychiatrists are medical doctors who have qualified in psychiatry.

Psychotherapy deals with the ways of helping people to overcome stress, emotional problems, relationship problems or troublesome habits.

Psychotherapy can be conducted in several different ways – individual, group, couple or family psychotherapy. However, all these treatments are based on talking to another person and sometimes doing things together. These are *talking treatments*, which include:

- cognitive behavioural therapy
- psychoanalytic therapy
- psychodynamic therapy
- humanistic and integrative psychotherapy
- systematic therapy
- hypno-psychotherapy
- experiential constructivist therapy.

A psychotherapist is usually a psychiatrist, psychologist or other mental health professional who has had further specialist training in psychotherapy.[4]

District nurse (DN)

A district nurse is a senior nurse similar to a ward sister in hospital, but with an added qualification like a *district nurse certificate*. The district nursing service is led by a district nurse and is run by the primary care trusts. As GPs are mainly responsible for meeting the medical needs in primary care, DNs are responsible for meeting the nursing needs in the community with the help of a team of dedicated workers. They take referrals from GPs, social services and hospitals.

Nursing, midwifery and health visiting make up the largest workforce in the NHS. They play a central role in a person's journey across sickness and health, home and hospital, birth and death. Like general practice, nursing in primary care has a long and proud tradition – providing expert care to individuals, families and communities in their homes, workplaces and schools and in surgeries. They provide the full spectrum of care from primary prevention through to specialist disease management and palliative care. Primary care services are delivered in the real everyday world where life is lived, where health is shaped and where the majority of care takes place.

Keeping pace with people's expectations, professional roles are changing with *extension of roles* and *skill mixing* and breaking down of the outdated organisational and professional barriers. To deliver the NHS Plan, nurses in primary care will need to be in the forefront of change and innovation. They will have:

- a greater voice in decision making
- greater skill mix and leadership opportunities
- a key role in delivering 24-hour first contact care across a range of settings
- opportunity to provide more secondary care in community settings
- extension of nursing roles including taking on some of the work currently done by GPs
- a major role in delivering National Service Frameworks.[3]

Social worker (SW)

Social work is a human rights discipline and social workers work with people to achieve social welfare, social justice and social inclusion, where that is sought by the individual. Social work is defined as:

A profession that promotes social changes, problem solving in human relationships and the empowerment and liberation of people to enhance well-being. Utilising theories of human behaviour and social systems, social work intervenes at the points where people interact with their environments. Principles of human rights and social justice are fundamental to social work.[2]

Social work is working towards a well-regulated workforce ensuring high standards of practice and an entry qualification of a four-year honours degree to qualify as a social worker.

Social workers have the responsibility to help individuals, families, groups and communities through the provision and operation of appropriate services and contributing to social planning. They work with, on behalf of or in the interests of people to enable them to deal with personal and social difficulties and obtain essential resources and services.

Some of the important areas where social workers play crucial roles are child protection, adults with incapacity (mental illness), domestic violence, young offenders and the criminal justice system.

Once an individual is referred to social services, he/she will be allocated a named social worker who will be responsible for assessing the needs of the person and making a care plan in partnership with the client, relatives and carers.

Under the current legislation, in the hospital set-up, once a patient (after being declared medically fit by the medical team) is referred to the social services (*section 2*), a social worker is expected to sort out the social issues within 3–4 days (except weekends). However, if they fail to do so, the hospital can issue a *section 5* notice. If the social services fail to respond within 24 hours of issuing a section 5, then the social services will be penalised. Social services will have to pay part of the cost for any extra day stay of the patient in the hospital (Delayed Discharge Act, DH).[3]

Sometimes social workers are asked by relatives, doctors, friends or neighbours to visit someone and to assess them under the Mental Health Act 1983. This is carried out by an *approved social worker (ASW)*.

An ASW is a social worker who has received specialist training and has been given responsibilities under the Mental Health Act 1983 to assess, when requested, whether a person needs to be detained in hospital. After assessing the patient, the ASW can arrange necessary support or voluntary hospital admission. However, if it is not possible because of the poor mental state of the patient, the ASW will consult with the person's GP and an approved psychiatrist and may arrange for detention in hospital for a period of assessment and/or treatment.[5]

Services

Depending on the type and degree of care needs, a variety of services can be offered:

- Home-care services.
- 'Care closer to home' services – the components are:
  - intermediate care
  - transitional care
  - hospital care at home.
- Continuing NHS healthcare.
- Respite care.
- Long-term care – the options are placement in:
  - sheltered accommodation, warden-controlled accommodation or elderly people's home
  - residential home
  - nursing home
  - EMI (elderly mentally ill) home.[1–3]

Home-care services

When an elderly person or couple cannot manage on their own and there are no responsible relatives or friends or neighbours available to help them, then the social services arrange help for them at home through social carers' input. Depending on the need social carers may visit from once a week up to a maximum of four times a day. The social carers help them in their cleaning, washing, preparing foods, shopping, collecting pension and other ADL. There is usually no carer available overnight.

Intermediate care (IC)

Intermediate care is defined as the care and support services that meet all of the following criteria:

- targeted at people who would otherwise face unnecessarily prolonged hospital stay or inappropriate admission to acute inpatient care, long-term residential care or continuing NHS inpatient care
- provided on the basis of a comprehensive assessment, resulting in a structured individual care plan that involves active therapy, treatment or opportunity for recovery
- have a planned outcome of maximising independence and typically enabling patients/users to resume living at home
- are time-limited, normally no longer than six weeks and frequently as little as 1–2 weeks or less and
- involve cross-professional working, with a single assessment framework, single professional records and shared protocols.

This service is available for individuals who require *a period of rehabilitation*, after illness or injury, to regain control and independence in their lives and this period can extend *up to a maximum of six weeks*. This service is usually provided in one of the designated wards in hospital or local residential or nursing home.

Service models

Intermediate care can encompass a range of services as follows:

- *Rapid response* – a service designed to prevent avoidable acute admissions by providing rapid assessment/diagnosis for patients referred from the GPs, A&E, NHS Direct or social services and if necessary rapid access on a 24-hour basis to short-term treatment, therapy or necessary support and care in the patient's own home.
- *Hospital at home* – an intensive support in the patient's own home, including investigations and treatments. This can be used either as a means of avoiding an acute admission or to enable earlier discharge from hospital.
- *Residential rehabilitation* – a short-term programme of therapy and enablement in a residential setting, such as community hospital, rehabilitation centre, nursing home or residential care home, for people who are medically stable but need a period of rehabilitation to enable them to regain sufficient physical functioning and confidence to return safely to their own home.
- *Supported discharge* – involves a short-term period of nursing and/or therapeutic support in a patient's home, typically with a contributory package of home-care and support services, to enable earlier transfer of their care from acute hospital and complete their rehabilitation and recovery at home.
- *Day rehabilitation* – a short-term programme of therapeutic support, provided at a day hospital or day centre. It may be used in conjunction with other forms of intermediate care. Day hospitals can also provide a one-stop rapid-response service with both specialist and multidisciplinary input.

In summary, IC service:

- facilitates timely discharge from hospital
- prevents inappropriate hospital admission
- provides intensive rehabilitation packages to promote independence and avoid long-term care/admission to residential and nursing homes.

IC service *does not provide*:

- longer-term rehabilitation
- convalescence
- respite care.

Referral criteria

Criteria for referral to IC service are as follows: The patient *must*:

- be over 16 years of age
- be resident and registered with a GP within that PCT boundary
- be a hospital inpatient at present or have attended A&E/required GP review at home within last 48 hours and a rehabilitation need identified
- have a level of memory recall and motivation that allow active participation in a rehabilitation programme
- have potential to improve physical functioning and/or regain independence
- have been seen by a therapist and a rehabilitation need identified
- give informed consent to receive the care.

Transitional care

This is another component of 'care closer to home' services and is also provided in one of the designated local residential or nursing homes for a *maximum period of up to six weeks*.
   The service *facilitates*:

- appropriate and early discharge from hospital
- reduction in number and length of delayed transfer of care
- support of patients requiring a passive recovery period (convalescence), either prior to possible rehabilitation or commencement of long-term care package.

The person must meet the following *criteria*:

- over the age of 55 years
- be resident and registered with a GP within that PCT boundary
- medically stable or declared fit to transfer
- currently a hospital inpatient
- has an *identified aim, outcome and exit route* at the point of referral.

Hospital care at home

Hospital at home service is an extension to the district nursing service by providing additional levels of support for patients at home. Referral to this service can usually be made 24 hours a day and seven days a week including bank holidays. This service is again available for a *maximum period of six weeks*, although it is mainly designed for patients who have a life expectancy of *less than two weeks*.

The patient should meet the following *criteria*:

- be resident and registered with a GP within that PCT boundary
- be over 16 years of age
- patient's health condition would necessitate admission to hospital without extra support
- patient's GP accepts medical responsibility
- patient's district nurse accepts nursing responsibility
- patient and carers consent to admission on to the scheme
- have care overseen by and receiving input from district nursing team.

Continuing NHS healthcare

One hundred per cent NHS-funded continuing healthcare is available for patients who meet certain criteria and can be of three types:

- continuing care, e.g. patient with severe stroke
- palliative care, e.g. patient with terminal cancers
- respite care, e.g. patient with dementia or stroke.

Continuing care and palliative care are usually provided in a nursing home set-up under the care of a hospital consultant, who reviews the patient regularly. Patients under the age of 65 years need special arrangements, as most nursing homes do not have the facilities to manage patients under 65.

Eligibility criteria for 100% NHS-funded continuing healthcare are subject always to the consideration of individual needs, which may need a formal health needs assessment.

Patients who meet one or more of the following criteria will be eligible.

- The nature or complexity or intensity or unpredictability of the person's healthcare needs requires regular supervision by a member of the NHS multidisciplinary team, such as a consultant, palliative care nurse/specialist, therapist or others.
- The person's needs require the routine use of specialist healthcare equipment under the supervision of NHS staff.
- The person has a rapidly deteriorating or unstable medical, physical or mental health condition and requires regular supervision by a member of the NHS multidisciplinary team.
- The person is in the final stage of a terminal illness, whereby medical opinion identifies that the patient is in a progressive state of decline and life expectancy is likely to be only days, weeks or months. Regard will be taken of the healthcare needs and choice of the patient and their family. No patient will be discharged from inpatient care without an individual assessment of their health needs and their expressed wishes taken into account.

Eligible without formal assessment – patients with one of the following conditions are eligible without any formal assessment:

- persons in a persistent vegetative state
- persons who are ventilator dependent
- persons in coma

- persons detained under sections 2, 3, 35, 36, 37 or 41 of the Mental Health Act 1983
- persons admitted compulsorily to hospital under the terms of the Mental Health Act or patients who would meet the requirements of the Act but are willing to be admitted voluntarily
- persons who are terminally ill with severe problems of symptom control.

Patients who do not meet any of the above criteria may still be entitled to have continuing care if the requirement to meet their healthcare needs goes beyond that which a local authority can be expected to provide pursuant to the obligations under section 21 of the National Assistance Act 1948.

Respite care

Respite refers to a short time of rest or relief. It allows the caregiver a break from day-to-day duties while the patient receives care from qualified individuals.

In the NHS, respite care must be approved by a hospital consultant and could be up to a maximum period of six weeks per year, usually as a two-week slot. However, outside the NHS it could be arranged privately through a number of agencies.

Patients with significant physical and/or mental disability for which they need regular supervision and help from a caregiver (spouse, partner, relative, neighbour, social carer or a volunteer) fulfil the criteria to receive NHS respite care. The following are examples of some eligible patients:

- patients with chronic disabling neurological conditions like stroke, Parkinson's disease, multiple sclerosis, motor neurone disease, encephalitis, etc.
- severe learning disability, Down's syndrome
- cerebral palsy
- dementia.

Respite care can be provided:

- occasionally or on a regular basis
- for part of the day, evening, overnight or days
- in a home, community organisation or residential facility.

There are several ways of providing respite care as follows.

- *in-home respite care* can provide the following types of services:
  - companion services – help with supervision, recreational activities and visiting
  - personal care services – assistance with bathing, dressing, toileting, exercising and other daily activities
  - homemaker services – help with housekeeping, shopping and meal preparation
  - skilled care services – help with medication and other medical services
- *adult day centres*
- *residential respite care* – in some specialised units in nursing homes or hospitals
- *informal respite care* – provided by a family member, close friend, neighbour or a volunteer
- *respite care for emergency situations*.

Respite care can be very beneficial for the health and well-being of the person providing care as well as the patient. It gives the caregiver the time and assistance needed to meet *personal needs* as well as *other responsibilities*. It can provide the patients:

- a chance to get out of the house, participate in enjoyable activities and socialise with others
- an opportunity to mix with others who are experiencing similar challenges
- time away in a safe environment with activities structured to meet their abilities and needs.

Long-term care

When someone cannot manage at home even with home helps, then he/she needs placement in one of the following residential facilities, depending on their degree of independence and intensity of care needs. All this care may be NHS funded or privately funded.

- *Sheltered accommodation, warden-controlled accommodation, elderly people's home care* – this is suitable for persons who are fully self-caring, but need companionship to help their loneliness and supervision of a warden in case they need any help.
- *Residential home care* – this is suitable for persons who mainly need help for their activities of daily living from a healthcare assistant/carer with minimal nursing needs. Residential home-care need is assessed by a *social worker* and this care is funded by social services.
- *Nursing home care* – this is suitable for persons who are largely nursing need dependent (e.g. patients on tube feeding, tracheostomy tube, etc.) and are usually fully dependent for their ADL. Nursing home-care need is assessed by a *social worker* along with a *nursing advisor* and this care is funded by the health services.
- *EMI home care* – patients who have significant psychiatric problems (e.g. psychosis, depression, dementia, etc.) need placement in homes with input from specially trained professionals (carers, nurses and psychiatrists) and these are known as EMI (elderly mentally ill) homes. EMI homes can be residential homes or nursing homes depending upon the need of the patient.

References

1   Byrne T and Padfield CF (1983) *Social Services (Made Simple Books)* (2e). Heinemann, Oxford.
2   Adams R, Dominelli L and Payne M (eds) (2002) *Social Work: themes, issues and critical debate* (2e). Palgrave, Basingstoke and New York.
3   Department of Health (DH) website: www.dh.gov.uk.
4   Allied Health Professionals – NHS Careers website: www.nhscareers.nhs.uk.
5   British Association of Social Workers website: www.basw.co.uk.

Section 4: Clinical governance, research and publications

- Clinical governance
- Medical research
- Medical publications

Chapter 13

Clinical governance

Clinical governance

Background

The need for quality-control measures in the NHS has been realised for a long time. The Bristol baby heart scandal in the late 1980s, however, shattered public confidence in NHS healthcare delivery. (Compared to other centres, a disproportionately large number of infants and children with congenital heart disease died after heart operations in the Bristol Cardio-Thoracic Centre and this was thought to be due to lack of necessary skills and competence of the concerned surgeons.) At the same time, it was revealed that the UK performs very poorly in the international league tables of cancer death rates and more than half of all cancer patients are not being referred to an appropriate cancer specialist despite the Calman-Hine recommendations, which heightened public dissatisfaction further. The Department of Health (DH) realised the urgent need for necessary steps to reform the NHS. The DH then started publishing a series of documents entitled 'White Paper' issues.

- The NHS White Paper *Working for Patients* (DH, 1989) addressed the issues of *clinical audit*.
- *The New NHS: modern, dependable* (DH, 1997) stated that the government will require every NHS trust to embrace the concept of clinical governance centring around the issues of quality and accountability at organisational and individual level.
- *A First Class Service: quality in the new NHS* (DH, 1998) defined *clinical governance*.[1]

Definition

A framework through which NHS organizations are accountable for continuously improving the quality of their services and safeguarding high standards of care by creating an environment in which excellence in clinical care will flourish.[1]

In other words, it is the involvement of clinicians and healthcare professionals to ensure quality and accountability in NHS healthcare delivery. The buzzwords are quality and accountability.

- *Quality* is what outcome you want and being sure you get it, every time, for as long as you want it.[2]
- *Accountability* is the responsibility of individuals or organisations for their actions and the ability to explain and justify their activity.

Principles of clinical governance (CG)

The principles of CG encompass a wide range of issues, of which the main ones are as follows:

- clinical audit
- clinical effectiveness monitoring
- *clinical risk management* – with adverse events being detected, openly investigated and lessons learnt
- evidence-based practice
- *staff development* – through lifelong learning and setting, maintaining and monitoring performance standards. Continuing medical education (CME), continuing professional development (CPD), record of in-training assessment (RITA), appraisal and revalidation are a few measures for staff development.[3]

Dimensions of clinical governance

- *Corporate accountability* – the accountable officer is the chief executive or the chair of the governing body of the NHS trust, who has the overall responsibility for clinical performance. A sub-committee led by a medical director or a chief nurse is responsible for the production of monthly reports of the trust board and a summary for inclusion in the annual report. NHS trusts produced their first clinical governance reports in Spring 2000.
- *Internal mechanisms* – include individual accountability, self and professional regulation, lifelong learning, CME and CPD.
- *External mechanisms* – include the following:
  - *Commission for Health Improvement (CHI)* – a statutory body which works like a watchdog. It provides national leadership to develop and disseminate clinical governance principles. It supports the NHS trusts to develop their local policies, visits the hospitals at regular intervals to assess the standard of care, find out any major defects in policy and helps to solve the problems. From 1 April 2004, all functions of CHI were taken over by the *Healthcare Commission*.
  - *National Institute for Clinical Excellence (NICE)* – responsible for producing and disseminating clinical guidelines based on relevant evidence of clinical and cost-effectiveness and associated clinical audit methodologies and information on good practice. On 1 April 2005, NICE joined with the Health Development Agency to become the new *National Institute for Health and Clinical Excellence (NIHCE, also to be known as NICE)*.
  - *National Service Frameworks (NSFs)* – develop protocols for management of various health-related problems, e.g. coronary heart disease, care of the elderly, etc.
  - *National Performance Framework (NPF)* – responsible for publishing local figures (e.g. death rates, complications rates, etc.), to the public.[3]

Clinical governance is to play an important role in reorganising the NHS and restoring public confidence in NHS healthcare delivery. It has increasingly become an integral part of our day-to-day clinical practice.

Clinical audit

Definition

Audit is a quality control tool used to assess, evaluate and improve our practice by comparing it with a set standard.

Medical audit is an integral part of our current medical practice. It is now compulsory for each and every NHS hospital to conduct monthly rolling half-day audits. In every NHS trust there is a defined audit department, an audit coordinator and a representative from each directorate *(directorate audit lead)* to organise regular audits. All elective activities (clinics, operations, etc.) are cancelled during audit sessions.

Audit cycle

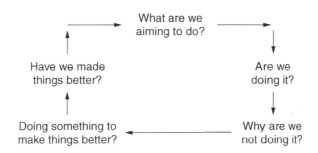

Figure 13.1 The audit cycle.

Steps in an audit

Step 1: Select a topic and determine specific parameters to be studied.
Step 2: Define your standards:
    a   *gold standard* – national or international guidelines
    b   *other standards* – local guidelines or accepted practice.
Step 3: The audit study – introduction/aims and objectives/methods/results/ discussion and conclusion.
Step 4: Highlight differences.
Step 5: Recommendations/develop coping strategies.
Step 6: Repeat the audit study – 'closing the audit loop'.

Types of audits

Audit studies can be *retrospective* or *prospective* and the purpose of an audit project may be:

- to compare with a known standard
- to set a standard where there is no established standard available
- re-audit to see the impact of recommendations of the original audit on clinical practice.

Organising an audit

Audits are conducted at local, regional or national level. If it is a regional or national audit, the audit methodology, criteria and proforma are provided by the centre coordinating the audit. In case of a local hospital audit the audit team will have to organise this with the help of the audit department.

The steps in organising an audit after selecting a particular topic are as follows:

- *Apply to the audit office* by filling out an *audit project proposal form*. The audit office will be able to tell you whether any audit on the same topic has been done in the recent past. This proposal form includes: audit title, name(s) of investigator(s), speciality, aims and objectives, sample identification, time period of sample, assessment method and outcome measures, and audit resources.
- *Ethics committee approval* – may be required if the audit study includes:
  - prospective study
  - clinical activities that are not part of routine practice
  - direct patient contact
  - likelihood to be submitted for publication
  - cross-site audit.
- *Data collection* – the methods used in audit studies include one of the following:
  - proforma – to collect data from case notes
  - computer data extraction
  - questionnaire
  - interview.
- *Data analysis and production of draft audit report.*

You have to specify what type of assistance you need from the audit department. A whole range of support is usually available from the audit department starting with identification of the study population, designing proformas/questionnaires, case-notes retrieval, database design, etc. to data analysis and presentation. However, all these (especially retrieval of a large number of case notes from the medical records department) are time consuming and you must plan well in advance. If you are planning to have some first-hand experience of an audit study in a short time period and to improve your CV, you may join in an already ongoing study or design a small study where you will need minimum or no support from the audit department.

Clinical effectiveness

Definition

Clinical effectiveness means 'doing the right thing, to the right people, at the right time and getting it right the first time'.

Measuring clinical effectiveness

Clinical effectiveness of any drug, intervention or policy is best assessed through randomised controlled trials (RCTs). NICE is responsible for assessing clinical effectiveness and producing guidelines for implementation in clinical practice. The stages of measuring clinical effectiveness are as follows:

- *Ask the right question* – which should be important, simple, specific, realistic, and focused on an area where change is possible.
- *Find the relevant evidence* – by searching published literature, expert committee's opinion, etc.
- *Weigh up the evidence* – as applicable in your particular situation.
- *Apply the evidence in practice* – by involving relevant people and overcoming barriers to application.
- *Evaluate the changes* – by making refinement to the application and continuing to monitor performance.
- *Apply the evidence in a wider context.*[4]

However, before applying these principles for considering a drug or intervention in managing a particular patient, the doctor should:

- identify for that particular patient the *ultimate objective of treatment* – cure, prevention of recurrence, limitation of functional disability, prevention of later complications, reassurance, palliation, symptomatic relief etc.
- select the *most appropriate treatment option (including the option of no treatment at all)* using all available evidence
- specify the *treatment target* – to help you to decide when to stop treatment, change its intensity or switch to some other form of treatment.

In the case of RCTs, the clinical effectiveness is measured with parameters like relative risk reduction (RRR), absolute risk reduction (ARR) and number needed to treat (NNT). For other forms of studies, relevant appropriate parameters (e.g. rate, odds ratio, etc.) are used.

Measuring clinical effectiveness takes into account both *clinical efficacy analysis* (as above) and also *economic analysis,* which helps to make choices in resource allocation. Economic analysis can be of four types as follows:

- *Cost minimisation analysis* – used when the effect of both interventions is known or assumed to be identical.
- *Cost effectiveness analysis* – used when the effect of the interventions can be expressed in term of one main outcome variable (e.g. mortality reduction).
- *Cost utility analysis* – used when the effect of interventions on health status has two or more important dimensions (e.g. benefits and side effects of drugs).
- *Cost benefit analysis* – used when it is desirable to compare an intervention for one condition with an intervention for another condition (e.g. to fund a heart transplantation programme or a stroke rehabilitation ward).[5]

Monitoring clinical effectiveness

Continuing evaluation is necessary to monitor clinical effectiveness. The methods used for this purpose are audit, assessment, appraisal and revalidation.

Clinical risk management

Definition

Clinical risk management is the process of detecting adverse events, investigating them openly and learning lessons from them to prevent further similar mishaps.

It is based on a framework designed to help identify the varied causes of:

- *system failure or latent human failures* – inadequate organisational policies or inappropriate decisions, which make the working environment more risky
- *equipment failure or inadequate/inappropriate defences* – faulty monitoring of equipment or procedures leading to the incident
- *active human failures* – which could be:
  - *errors* (making slips, lapses or mistakes) – mistakes can be *rule based* (e.g. good use of a bad rule or bad use of a good rule) or *knowledge based* (e.g. bias or wrong mind-setting) or
  - *violations* – breaking or violating rules or protocols, which may be a routine practice, a personal failure or a necessity in some particular situation.

Adverse event, near miss and potential incident

An *adverse event or incident* is defined as 'an unintended injury that was caused by medical management and that resulted in measurable disability'. In a broader sense an adverse incident is 'any occurrence which is not consistent with the routine care of the patient or the routine operation of the institution'.

A *near miss* is defined as 'an occurrence, which but for luck or skilful management would in all probability have become an adverse incident'.

The National Patient Safety Agency (NPSA) is now advocating a proactive approach for looking for a *potential incident*, rather than a reactive approach of analysing an adverse event which has actually happened. Clinical risk management can thus be targeted at three levels:

- adverse event – which has actually happened
- near miss – which almost happened
- potential incident – which could have happened.

Hierarchy of risk management

The *chief executive* has the ultimate accountability in the trust to implement the principles of clinical governance, of which clinical risk management is an important one. The final decision on claim management is taken by the chief executive officer in consultation with the medical director, a non-executive director and the director of finance.

The *medical director* is the chairman of the Risk Management Committee and the Incident and Claims Review Committee. In consultation with the director of nursing and the risk manager, the medical director implements policies to provide a systematic and strategic approach to the management of all clinical risks within the trust.

The *risk manager* helps to design, implement and coordinate the trust's clinical risk management programme. He is responsible for implementation of a hospital-wide risk education and prevention programme, an induction programme in risk management for all new employees, and development and maintenance of the adverse incident reporting system with agreement from the Risk Management Committee.

Risk indicators

A major component of the management of clinical risk is an agreed system for the reporting of clinically related patient incidents and near misses. One of the duties of the Risk Management Committee is to produce and review a list of *risk indicators*.

Some of the risk indicators are *non-specific* and some are specific *speciality based* (e.g. surgical, obstetric, paediatric, anaesthetic, psychiatric, etc.). Examples of a few risk indicators are misdiagnosis, medication error, failure to act upon abnormal pathology or imaging results, falls leading to severe injury or fracture, development of grade 3/4 pressure sores while on ward, surgery on wrong patient or wrong side, unplanned removal of an organ during surgery, neonatal or maternal death, delayed diagnosis of important congenital malformations, etc.

An injured patient usually wants to understand the truth of what happened and to feel that steps have been taken to prevent recurrence. An honest explanation of the events and an early apology, without necessarily admitting liability, often prevents future litigation. The National Patient Safety Agency (NPSA) has launched a campaign called *'Being Open'*, urging doctors to apologise for errors they make, and it says 'an apology is not an admission of liability and will make patients less likely to make a litigation claim'. The Medical Director of NPSA, Professor Sir John Lilleyman, commented that 'Being Open' is the best policy and reinforced his belief that 'the medical profession requires a clear and unequivocal steer about the thorny issue of apologising and explaining what happened to a patient'.[6]

Incident reporting and disciplinary action

Clinical risk management depends on effective and regular reporting of adverse incidents and near misses. Every effort must be made to avoid cover-ups of adverse incidents, mistakes and near misses. To implement an effective incident-reporting system, the trust will have to establish a *no-blame culture*. The chief executive should ensure that no disciplinary action will result from reporting incidents, mistakes or near misses, unless the behaviour is criminal, is malicious, constitutes gross misconduct or deviates from the trust's published policy.

The system of reporting adverse events must be simple, straightforward and understood by all staff. The use of a *single incident-reporting form* will promote compliance. It is necessary to introduce an *explicit flow path* for the incident forms to ensure that incidents are all reviewed and graded by the clinical risk manager before entry into the database and that the appropriate forms are then received by the health and safety, occupational health and other relevant departments.

Principal objectives

Clinical risk management aims to achieve four main objectives as follows:

- Early identification of latent failures and defence inadequacies, so that managers can act to remedy the situation before any accident occurs.
- Prompt incident reporting allows the risk manager to collect relevant records, necessary documents and witness statements relating to incidents soon after the accident, which helps defending the case to a great extent.
- Early warning of possible claims allows up-to-date evidence to be used by the trust to consider whether to settle or fight a possible claim or resolve a clinical complaint. Honesty with the patient and a move to an early equitable settlement (where appropriate) are usually better for the patient, the staff involved and the hospital.
- Early and structured investigation of the adverse incident helps to find the underlying failures or deficiencies and enables the hospital to learn lessons, so that safety can be enhanced and further accidents prevented.[7]

Some other definitions

- *Clinical guidelines* are defined as 'systematically developed statements to help clinicians and clients in making decisions about care'.[1]
- *Clinical protocols* are defined as 'locally adapted versions of the broad statements of good practice contained in national guidelines'.[1]

Evidence-based medicine

Definition

This is a buzzword and there is a journal by the same title. Essentially, it means the conscientious and judicious use of the current and best available evidence from clinical research for the management of individual patients.

Research-based evidence has to be used in the context of available clinical expertise and patients' preference.

Strength of evidence

- *1++*: Evidence obtained from high-quality meta-analyses, systematic reviews of RCTs, or RCTs with a very low risk of bias.
- *1+*: Evidence obtained from well-conducted meta-analyses, systematic reviews, or RCTs with a low risk of bias.
- *1-*: Evidence obtained from meta-analyses, systematic reviews, or RCTs with a high risk of bias.
- *2++*: Evidence obtained from high-quality systematic reviews of case control or cohort studies; or high-quality case control or cohort studies with a very low risk of confounding or bias and a high probability that the relationship is causal.

- 2^+: Evidence obtained from well-conducted case control or cohort studies with a low risk of confounding or bias and a moderate probability that the relationship is causal.
- 2^-: Evidence obtained from case control or cohort studies with a high risk of confounding or bias and a significant risk that the relationship is not causal.
- 3: Evidence obtained from non-analytic studies, e.g. case reports, case series.
- 4: Evidence obtained from expert committee reports or opinions.

Grades of recommendations

- A: Requires at least one systematic review, meta-analysis or RCT rated 1^{++} and directly applicable to the target population; *or*, a body of evidence consisting principally of studies rated 1^+, directly applicable to the target population, and demonstrating overall consistency of results.
- B: Requires a body of evidence including studies rated as 2^{++}, directly applicable to the target population, and demonstrating overall consistency of results; *or* extrapolated evidence from studies rated as 1^{++} or 1^+.
- C: Requires a body of evidence including studies rated as 2^+, directly applicable to the target population, and demonstrating overall consistency of results; *or* extrapolated evidence from studies rated as 2^{++}.
- D: Requires evidence level 3 or 4; *or* extrapolated evidence from studies rated as 2^+.[8]

Implementing evidence into practice

Implementing research-based evidence into clinical practice may be difficult and time consuming, as sometimes it may require health professionals to change their long-held beliefs and patterns of behaviour. The visible and measurable part of our professional practice is only the *tip of the iceberg*, which rests on the submerged broad base composed of our experiences, knowledge, values, attitudes, beliefs, assumptions and expectations. To get evidence into practice and bring about a change we have to:

- consider individual beliefs, attitudes and knowledge likely to influence the behaviour of the concerned professionals and managers
- identify factors likely to influence the proposed changes
- plan appropriate interventions to overcome potential barriers
- be aware of the important influences in the organisational, economic and community environments
- motivate people to tackle the changes
- provide adequate resources
- incorporate monitoring and evaluation systems from the beginning
- implement the change and find ways to maintain and reinforce the new practices.

A recent review by the Cochrane Effective Practice and Organisation of Care Group (EPOC) revealed the common underlying reasons for the gap between evidence and practice and the degree of effectiveness of various methods used to implement evidence into practice.

Reasons for the gap between evidence and practice include:

- lack of knowledge and/or lack of confidence
- fear of legal or patient pressure or loss of income
- lack of physical skill
- inadequate resources
- pressure of work
- old habits.

The degree of effectiveness of various methods is as follows:

- *Consistently effective methods* – educational outreach visits (academic detailing), reminder or prompts issued at the time of consultation, interactive educational meetings, practical hands-on education and use of locally produced and owned protocols.
- *Sometimes effective methods* – audit and feedback, patient-led/mediated strategies (e.g. information leaflets) and rules and incentives.
- *Little or no effect* – was found with didactic educational meetings or distribution of printed guidelines and protocols.[5]

Staff development

Introduction

The fundamental aim of clinical governance is to provide a first-class service with a high standard of care to the patients. To provide a high standard of care healthcare professionals should be well trained and up to date in their knowledge and skills, which in turn depends on continuing education and training and monitoring. One of the key objectives of implementation of clinical governance in the NHS is to establish the cultures of *learning*, *research* and *development* and encourage *evaluation* and *feedback*.

The dynamics of provision of healthcare is based on three systems: *education and training*, *service* and *research and development*. The education and training system is designed, run and monitored by Postgraduate Deanery and Education and Training Consortia in close cooperation with professional and statutory bodies like the Royal Colleges, staff training committees (STCs), General Medical Council (GMC), etc.

The academic learning is provided via a university-based system whereas the practical application of that academic learning is operated through the NHS trusts and general practices. The funding for education and training partly comes from the health authority allocations via three levies: *Service Increment for Teaching (SIFT)*, *Medical and Dental Education Levy (MADEL)* and *Non-Medical Education and Training Levy (NMET)*. SIFT is a levy which funds the additional costs to the NHS of supporting the clinical teaching of undergraduate medical students. MADEL covers part of the basic salaries of doctors in training and the local costs for the facilities for postgraduate medical and dental education, such as maintenance of postgraduate centres and libraries, costs of study leave, etc. NMET covers the costs of the education and training of professions other than doctors and dentists.[7]

To keep up to date in knowledge and skills a professional will have to continue lifelong learning, i.e. from cradle to grave of his/her professional career. This is called continuing medical education (CME) or continuing professional development (CPD).

Continuing professional development (CPD)

Continuing professional development is defined as 'a process of lifelong learning for all individuals and teams which meets the needs of patients, and delivers the health outcomes and health priorities of the NHS and enables professionals to expand and fulfil their potential'.[9]

This continuing education and training should be implemented at individual level, team level and organisational level and it should be multiprofessional as well as uniprofessional. CPD needs to be sensitive to individual and organisational needs. However, as these two needs are not always the same, there may be conflict between the service needs and professional aspirations.

The CPD measures at individual level include reading journals and textbooks, attending meetings, seminars and courses, presenting in meetings and research and publications.

Personal development planning is an important part of the CPD cycle. This includes a detailed set of *work objectives* and detailed *training and development objectives*, linked to work objectives; both should be mutually agreed with the individual's manager. They have to be supported by success criteria, deadlines for achieving the objectives and dates for reviewing progress in meeting those objectives.

All consultants and non-consultant career grade doctors are expected to maintain a *CPD diary* through the *CPD register* in their respective colleges (e.g. RCP London). A specialist registrar is to start a CPD diary from the final year of training.[9]

Record of in-training assessment (RITA)

Record of in-training assessment is a formal documentation of the regular assessment of the HO, SHO and specialist registrars in their training records. It is done by the educational supervisor and incorporates record of *core skills training, medical training, educational activities and appraisal.*

The trainees should have their first meeting with the educational supervisor during the first month of the post to set educational objectives for the period in which they will be working in the unit and to clarify their long-term aims. It is advisable that the educational supervisor meets the trainee informally midway in the post to check on progress. There will be a final assessment with appraisal at the end of the post.

RITA is the process of measuring or describing competence and performance against defined criteria based on relevant content. It is an opportunity to check progress regularly (usually annually) against the core curriculum. This is intended to provide support and guidance to trainees and trainers, and to assess the requirements of the post and whether the required standards are being achieved. It provides feedback from trainee to educational supervisor on the quality of the post and training programmes. Essentially RITA determines career progression and is entirely for the benefit of the trainee.

At specialist registrar grade, RITA has been designed to fulfil the following functions:

- to provide a simple and effective mechanism for recording and managing trainees' progress towards their training goal and through the SpR grade
- to provide a device which enables assessment, however it is to be carried out
- to provide a framework to link the responsibilities of the Royal Colleges and faculties for assessment to those of the postgraduate deans
- to enable assessment of out-of-programme clinical work and
- to provide a final statement of the trainee's successful completion of the training programme.

There are seven forms which comprise RITA, each contained on a single page:

- *Form A*: *Core Information on the Trainee* – must be completed before the doctor is registered in the training programme.
- *Form B*: *Changes to Core Information* – this must be completed annually if there is any change of core information given in Form A.
- *Form C*: *Record of Satisfactory Progress within the Specialist Registrar Grade* – it is essential to permit progress through the grade and normally required annually.
- *Form D*: *Recommendation for Targeted Training (Stage 1 of 'Required Additional Training')* – allows conditional progress through the grade and a further Form C will be required to progress at the end of the stipulated period of required additional training.
- *Form E*: *Recommendation for Intensified Supervision/Repeated Experience (Stage 2 of 'Required Additional Training')* – requires that part or all of the period of training under review should be repeated and a further Form C will be required to progress at the end of this stipulated period of required additional training.
- *Form F*: *Record of Out-of-Programme Experience* – is essential to retain the validity of an NTN (national training number) or VTN (vocational training number) and to inform the postgraduate dean of out-of-programme progress.
- *Form G*: *Final Record of Satisfactory Progress* – this form is used instead of a Form C in the final assessment. It is essential for the deanery to issue in order to enable the relevant college or faculty to recommend to the STA (specialist training authority) the award of a CCST (Certificate of Completion of Specialist Training).

The maximum number of forms that can be completed at any one review is two – a Form B (if required) and one of the Forms C, D, E, F or G.[10]

Appraisal

Appraisal is a process being introduced by the Department of Health for doctors working in the NHS. The aim is to give doctors regular feedback on past performance and continuing progress and to identify education and development needs for their career development.

Appraisal is:

A professional process of constructive dialogue in which the doctor being appraised has a formal structured opportunity to reflect on his/her work and consider how his/her effectiveness might be improved.

A positive process to give someone feedback on their performance, to chart their continuing progress and to identify the development needs. It is a forward looking process, essential for the developmental and educational planning needs of an individual.

The appraisal process is the vehicle through which the GMC revalidation requirements will be delivered. To this end appraisal discussions must be sufficiently broad to cover the essential requirements of revalidation.

It is the responsibility of the chief executive to ensure that consultants' appraisal takes place regularly and annually.

Appraisers must be adequately trained in the process of appraisal. The clinical director is usually responsible for appraisal of consultants and non-consultant career grade doctors (NCCGs) in his/her directorate. The clinical director and if needed other consultants should be appraised by directorate lead consultants or other trained appraisers appointed to an approved appraiser 'bank'.

Appraisal became a contractual requirement for consultants since 1 April 2001 and for GP principals since 1 April 2002. Appraisal for other groups of doctors – including non-consultant career grades, public health doctors, doctors in training and locum doctors – was introduced towards the end of 2003.[1,11–14]

The appraisal process consists of discussion on the following issues:

- details of current job plan and activities
- future personal development plan
- good medical care (evidence – current job plan/work programme, annual caseload/workload, list of audit works, etc.)
- maintaining good medical practice (evidence – up-to-date CPD certificate, certificate of attendance at national or international conference/meeting/courses, etc.)
- working relationship with colleagues (evidence – 360° assessment report, now known as multi-source feedback or MSF)
- relations with patients (evidence – 360° assessment report or MSF)
- teaching and training (evidence – feedback from teaching sessions [evaluation forms], letter from college tutor, etc.)
- probity and Health (needs evidence if there is any problem)
- management activity.

See Table 13.1 for some differences between appraisal and assessment.

Table 13.1 Differences between appraisal and assessment

Assessment	Appraisal
Looks back	Looks back to look forward
One way	Two way
Pre-defined criteria/external standards	Discussion
Pass/fail	Building
Right/wrong	Improving

Revalidation

Revalidation is a process whereby doctors will have to demonstrate regularly to the GMC that they are fit to practise medicine. Doctors who are successful will be granted a licence to practise. Doctors who choose not to participate in revalidation will be able to stay on the register without the entitlement to exercise the privileges currently associated with registration. If concerns are raised about a doctor's fitness to practise during the revalidation process, he/she will be referred to the GMC's Fitness to Practise procedures.

It is the responsibility of every doctor to be able to show the GMC that he/she has followed the principles set out in *Good Medical Practice* which are relevant to his/her speciality and practice. Revalidation is the combination of the doctors doing it and the GMC confirming the continuity of their licence to practise.

There are two main routes to revalidation:

- *the appraisal route* – to use this route to revalidation, you will have to show the GMC that, during the revalidation period, you have worked in a managed environment and have participated in an annual appraisal system
- *the independent route* – to use this route, you have to show the GMC that you are adopting the principles of *Good Medical Practice* within your professional practice and undertaking appropriate CME or CPD.

Your licence to practise will be withdrawn in the following situations:

- you tell the GMC that you no longer want it
- you do not pay the appropriate fee
- you do not take part in the revalidation process when the GMC ask you to, or
- a Fitness to Practise panel directs that your registration should be suspended or erased.

The GMC was supposed to grant a licence to practise to all doctors on the register by the end of 2004, to take effect from 1 January 2005, after which no doctor will be able to practise without a licence.[15] The revalidation process was due to start from April 2005 and to be repeated every five years.

Sir Graeme Catto, President of the GMC, said that: 'the whole purpose of revalidation is to create public confidence that all licensed doctors are up to date and fit to practise'.[16] However, considering a few serious issues arising from the *Shipman Inquiry's fifth report*, the GMC agreed to postpone the introduction of revalidation until a review (led by the Chief Medical Officer of England, Sir Liam Donaldson) has been completed. (*Dr Harold Shipman was a homicidal psychopath GP from Greater Manchester, who killed more than 15 (maybe up to 250) of his vulnerable patients over a couple of decades of his practice in the late twentieth century with high-dose opiates.*) The chairwoman of the inquiry, Dame Janet Smith, expressed in her fifth report, *Safeguarding Patients: lessons from the past, proposals for the future*, that 'the public cannot properly have confidence that a doctor who has been revalidated is "up to date and fit to practise"'.[17] She also made a few recommendations for revalidation which include:

- each doctor to prepare a folder of evidence with compulsory elements such as prescribing data, records of complaints or concerns, professional development activities, a patient satisfaction questionnaire, results of clinical audit and significant event audits

- assessment of each folder by a panel including a lay person
- a video recording of the doctor in consultation with patients to be provided
- tougher appraisal that might be rated as 'pass' or 'fail'
- a knowledge test
- positive certification at the end of the first stage of revalidation that a doctor is fit to practise; if not achieved, this would lead immediately to further GMC scrutiny.

Sir Liam Donaldson is reviewing the whole situation with the help of the BMA and Royal Colleges, keeping in mind the importance of the public having confidence in the revalidation system and also of the need to have a system that is practical for working doctors.[11,14–17]

References

1 Department of Health website: www.dh.gov.uk.
2 Lilley R (1999) *Making Sense of Clinical Governance: a workbook for NHS doctors, nurses and managers* (1e). Radcliffe Medical Press, Oxford.
3 Wilson J and Tingle J (1998) Clinical governance. *British Journal of Nursing*. **7** (16): 987–8.
4 Chambers R and Wakley G (2000) *Making Clinical Governance Work for You* (1e). Radcliffe Medical Press, Oxford.
5 Greenhalgh T (2001) *How to Read a Paper: the basics of evidence based medicine* (2e). BMJ Books, London.
6 National Patient Safety Agency website: www.npsa.nhs.uk.
7 Lugon M and Secker-Walker J (1999) *Clinical Governance: making it happen* (1e). Royal Society of Medicine Press, London and Illinois.
8 Scottish Intercollegiate Guidelines Network (SIGN): www.sign.ac.uk.
9 Federation of the Royal Colleges of Physicians of the UK (2002) *CPD for UK Physicians*. February. Federation of the Royal Colleges of Physicians of the UK, London.
10 NHS Executive (1998) *A Guide to Specialist Registrar Training*. February. NHSE, London and Leeds.
11 General Medical Council website: www.gmc-uk.org.
12 DH and GMC join forces (2002) Appraisal and revalidation. *GMC News*. April.
13 Royal College of Physicians (2002) Consultant appraisal in the NHS: guidance for appraisees and appraisers. *RCP – Education and Training*. February.
14 General Medical Council (2003) Appraisal and revalidation: making revalidation work. *GMC News*. June.
15 General Medical Council (2003) A licence to practise and revalidation. *GMC News*. April.
16 General Medical Council (2005) Revalidation and licensing on hold. *GMC News*. February.
17 British Medical Association (2005) Revalidation revisited. *BMA News*. 19 February: 12.

Chapter 14

Medical research

Definition

Research is a systematic and rigorous investigation of materials undertaken to discover/establish facts or relationships and reach conclusions using scientifically sound methods. It describes the processes and develops explanatory concepts ultimately to contribute to a scientific body of knowledge.

Why research?

- To know *'what is the right thing to do?'* and hence to practise evidence-based medicine.
- To become research literate (to read, write and understand papers).
- To satisfy the requirement of academic career progression.

How is research related to audit and clinical governance?

- *Clinical research* – answers 'What is the right thing to do?'
- *Clinical audit* – answers 'Are we doing the thing right?'
- *Clinical governance* – ensures that the thing is being done right.

Research vs audit

Research and audit have much in common and sometimes the distinction between the two is not clear to healthcare professionals. However, there are a number of fundamental differences between these two disciplines. Sometimes, larger projects may contain elements of both audit and research.

Research can identify areas for audit, whereas audit can pinpoint areas where research evidence is lacking and also helps in dissemination of evidence-based practice. Thus, clinical audit can be legitimately viewed as the final stage of a good clinical research programme.

We have to ask *three basic questions* to decide whether a proposed project is an audit or research:

1 Is the purpose of the project to improve the quality of care in the local setting?
2 Will the project involve measuring practice against set standards?
3 Does the project involve anything being done to the patients which would not have been part of their normal routine management?

If the answers to the first two questions are 'Yes' and the answer to the third question is 'No', then the proposed project is an audit; otherwise it is some form of research.

The *similarities* between research and audit can be summarised as follows:[1]

- Both involve answering a specific question relating to quality of care.
- Both can be carried out either prospectively or retrospectively.
- Both involve careful sampling, questionnaire design and analysis of findings.
- Both activities should be professionally led.

The differences between research and audit can be summarised as in Table 14.1.

Table 14.1 Differences between research and audit

Research	Audit
Creates new knowledge and determines what the best practice is	Answers the question 'Are we following the best practice?'
Based on a hypothesis	Measures against a set standard
Usually of large scale and carried out over prolonged period	Usually of small scale and short duration
May involve experiment or new treatment on patients	Usually does not involve doing anything to the patients beyond normal routine clinical management
Based on scientifically valid sample size (except in pilot study)	Sample size estimation is not always scientifically based
Extensive statistical analysis of data is routine	Simple statistical analysis of data is the usual norm
Results are generalisable and hence publishable	Results are usually relevant to local setting, but sometimes publishable in the interest of the wider audience
Always requires ethical approval	Rarely requires ethical approval

Broad fields of medical research

The field of medical research is broadly divided into the following five categories:

- *Therapy/intervention* – includes studying the efficacy of an intervention or therapy (e.g. surgical procedure or drugs).
- *Diagnosis* – tests the validity and reliability of a new diagnostic test by comparing with a gold standard test.
- *Screening* – assesses the efficacy of a test carried out in a large population in detecting a disease at a pre-symptomatic stage by comparing with a gold standard test.
- *Prognosis* – studies the short-term and long-term outcome of a condition.
- *Causation* – studies the causal relationship between exposure and development of an illness.[2]

Types of research studies

Research studies are primarily of two types as follows:

- *Quantitative research* – expresses mainly the investigators' viewpoint.
- *Qualitative research* – expresses mainly the subjects' viewpoint. Qualitative research methods are particularly suitable for *primary care* research because of:
  - their holistic approach
  - small numbers are acceptable and
  - their focus on people as social beings rather than as physiological systems.

Research studies can again be classified into two types:

1 *Primary research* – the studies report research first hand and can be one of the following:
  a *experimental studies:*
    - experiments on animals or volunteers in artificial and controlled environments
    - randomised controlled trials
    - (non-randomised) controlled clinical trials
  b *observational studies:*
    - cohort studies
    - case control studies
    - cross-sectional studies
    - surveys
    - case reports.
2 *Secondary research* – the studies summarise and draw conclusions from primary research studies and can be as follows:
  a *overviews:*
    - simple review – simply summarises the primary studies
    - systematic review – an overview of primary studies, which is conducted according to an explicit, predefined and reproducible methodology
    - meta-analysis – the statistical synthesis of numerical results of several primary studies which addressed the same clinical question
  b *economic analysis*
  c *decision analysis*
  d *guidelines development.*[2,3]

Research study designs

Study design means a chosen method of collecting information necessary to answer a particular research question. Choosing a particular study design involves decisions on the following:

- whether to intervene actively or simply describe what is observed *(experimental vs observational)*
- the timing for collecting information on exposure and outcome *(prospective vs retrospective* or *longitudinal vs cross-sectional)*
- the choice of control *(parallel group vs crossover study)*
- randomisation *(randomised vs non-randomised)*

Table 14.2 Choosing a research study design

Field of research	Type of study	Parameters of interest	Measures of effect
Therapy/intervention	Randomised controlled trials	Absolute risk/ relative risk	ARR/RRR/NNT
Diagnosis/ screening	Cross-sectional study	Sensitivity/ specificity/ accuracy	Odds ratio
Prognosis	Cohort study	Rate/risk/odds	Rate/risk ratio or difference, odds ratio
Causation	Cohort study Case control study Case reports	Rate/risk/odds Absolute risk	Rate, risk or odds ratio, relative risk
Incidence	Cohort study	Rate	Rate ratio/ Risk ratio
Prevalence	Cross-sectional study	Odds	Risk/odds ratio

- blinding *(single blind or double blind vs open)* and
- required *sample size*, etc.

Selection of an appropriate study design is vital to the ultimate success of the whole lengthy process involved in a research study. Depending on *what clinical question the study is going to answer*, we have to choose an appropriate study design from the above list. Table 14.2 shows a rough guide to choosing an appropriate study design based on which broad field of research the study is addressing, along with parameters of interest and measures of effect (which will be discussed in detail in Section 5, 'Medical statistics').[2]

A few common terms, used in various research study designs, are explained under the heading 'Research glossary' below.[2,4,5]

Research glossary

- *Experimental studies* – the investigator can intervene actively and has some control over the study, so the events are manipulated to some extent.
- *Observational studies* – follow the natural course of events without any active intervention. These studies could be:
  - *analytical* – where an exposure has been assigned (e.g. case control study, cohort study and cross-sectional study) or
  - *descriptive* – where the natural course of events is observed and the outcome reported (e.g. survey).
- *Longitudinal studies* – investigate a process over a period of time, which could be prospective or retrospective (e.g. cohort study, case control studies, etc.).
- *Cross-sectional studies* – observations are made at a single point of time. These

are observational studies, which could be descriptive or analytical as above. The main outcome measure is prevalence, either point prevalence or period prevalence. They are *quick and cheap*, but do not give any information about the causation or past of the disease (e.g. surveys, prevalence studies, etc.).

- *Prospective studies* – are also known as *follow-up studies* in which the data on *exposure* are collected first, and the subjects are followed up over a period of time for the development of a given condition or *outcome*. They give us valuable information on exposure, disease trend and impacts of the intervention in question. However, they need large samples, time and money. Examples are cohort study, clinical trials, etc.
- *Retrospective studies* – are observational studies in which information on *outcome* (presence or absence of disease) is collected first, and the subjects are subsequently investigated for possible past *exposure* or a *risk factor* of interest. Examples are case control studies and rarely some cohort studies. These studies are usually quick and cheap, but the most important disadvantage of these studies is incomplete or non-comparable information on all study subjects.
- *Case control studies* – are usually retrospective studies, which start at the end point and go backwards in time to try to identify risk factors which the subjects (known as *cases*) might have been exposed to in the past. The results are compared with a group of subjects who don't have the disease in question (known as *controls*, commonly selected through some form of *matching*). These studies are suitable for investigating rare diseases, need relatively small sample sizes and are relatively quick and cheap. However, precise definition of cases and choice of suitable control group are the most difficult parts in designing a case control study. They are also prone to various *biases* (selection bias, observer bias, recall bias, responder bias, etc.).
- *Cohort studies* – may be prospective or retrospective. Prospective cohort studies are usually concerned with the *aetiology* of a disease or with the *prognosis* of those already suffering from a disease. They follow a group of individuals with a particular risk factor, exposure or disease (known as a *cohort*) over some period of time, until some *end point* (usually *death* or development of the *disease* of interest) is reached. These studies need long-term follow-up, large sample sizes and are very expensive.

  Retrospective cohort studies are rare, but relatively quick, cheap and suitable for conditions with long latency periods. However, they have the usual disadvantages of retrospective studies.
- *Crossover or parallel group study* – the commonest approach used in clinical trials is *parallel design*, in which the new treatment is given to one group (the *treatment* or *test* group) and at the same time the conventional treatment or a placebo is given to a second group (the *control* group).

  Crossover design is a less frequently used approach in which one half of the subjects are given one treatment and the other half are given the second treatment. After a short washout period to prevent any carry-over effects, the two groups then swap treatments. As each subject in this study design acts as his/her own control, it needs a smaller sample size. However, it is not suitable for conditions that can be cured and a high dropout rate is a common problem.
- *Factorial design* – a study design that enables us to investigate the effects of multiple independent variables (both separately and combined) on a given outcome. For example: assessment of effects of two treatments A (aspirin) and

B (blood pressure lowering) in prevention of stroke. Here in a 2×2 contingency table, we can compare these treatments with each other and with a control simultaneously. The patients are divided into four groups – patients receiving control (or no) treatment, A only, B only, or both A and B. This design helps to study the interaction between A and B as well. However, this design is not commonly used in clinical trials.

- *Controls* – subjects used in comparative studies to act as the standard against which new treatments or interventions are to be tested or the risk connected with a particular exposure is evaluated. Controls can be concurrent or historical and they may be a different group of subjects or the same group as in a crossover study.
- *Bias* – the systematic error which leads to results that are consistently wrong in one or other direction. When bias is present in an investigation, the validity of the results will be open to question. There are different types of biases:
  - *selection bias* – randomisation is the best way to avoid it
  - *information biases* – due to systematic errors in measuring *exposures* or *outcome*, which result in misclassification. They include surveillance bias, recall bias, performance bias, attrition bias, etc. *Blinding* is the way to minimise this bias
  - *confounding bias* – the error that occurs when groups being compared in a study are different with regard to important *risk* or *prognostic factors* other than the factor under investigation. In the *randomised controlled trials*, these confounding errors are minimised or avoided by making groups comparable in relation to known and unknown prognostic factors. However, confounding remains a main problem in *case control studies*
  - *publication bias* – the type of bias that arises due to selective publication in medical journals of only those articles that report *statistically significant* positive results. Given that the statistical significance is not synonymous with *quality*, *validity* or *clinical significance*, this practice can cause studies of poor quality and misleading results to have much greater impact on clinical and policy decisions than they merit. Also, good studies which have conclusively demonstrated a lack of treatment effect or lack of association (i.e. a negative result) may never get to be published as their importance is often underestimated. *Systematic* and *exhaustive review* of all published and unpublished studies on the particular subject of interest is the way to avoid this bias.
- *Blinding* (or masking) – used in the context of *clinical trials*, whenever the participants (*single blind*) or both the participants and the researchers (*double blind*) are kept unaware of the treatment given or received. This avoids occurrence of observer and respondent biases (*information biases*). Placebos act as blinding measures in many trials.
- *Randomisation* – a process of allocating patients or participants to the alternative treatments or interventions in a *clinical trial*, with a view to produce comparable treatment groups in respect to important prognostic factors and thus to minimise the *selection bias*. There are several methods of randomisation as follows:
  - *simple randomisation* – the simplest way is to use a coin or a six-sided die or a table of random numbers (similar to using a ten-sided die). The main problem with this method is that it cannot ensure that at the end of recruitment there will be equal numbers of patients in two groups

- *blocked randomisation* – the allocation procedure is organised in such a way that equal numbers of cases are allocated to two groups. As an example, we can use a block of four containing two from each group (T = test group, C = control group) in all possible combinations (e.g. TCTC, TTCC, TCCT, CTCT, CCTT and CTTC)
- *stratified block randomisation* – here the confounding variables like patients' age, sex, etc. are taken into account to minimise selection bias further. Stratification can be made for any confounding variable, but it is usually advisable not to go beyond two variables. The method of balancing a large number of strata is known as *minimisation*.
  Randomisation and blinding in a study allow all subjects to have equal opportunity to be assigned to either group and minimise bias, thereby assuring that any difference observed between the groups is purely due to chance. Remote randomisation (telephone/internet) and double blinding are the best options.
- *Intention to treat analysis* – in this study the patients are analysed in the groups to which they were randomised, ignoring the fact that some patients may drop out or be withdrawn from the trial. This approach minimises the bias arising from these situations.
- *Randomised controlled trial (RCT)* – is the gold standard study design in medical research, but sometimes may not be feasible ethically or may not be appropriate. It has got the strength of having minimum bias, most precise estimation of effect and best quality evidence (level 1), which can change clinical practice. The sample population is randomly assigned to an experimental arm and a control arm and the outcome of intervention is compared between the two. An RCT utilises the following basic statistical concepts:
  - *independence* – the outcome of one event does not influence the outcome of any other
  - *randomness* – even though the individual outcomes are uncertain, there is a regular distribution of outcomes in a large number of repetitions
  - *law of large numbers* – with increasing number of observations (sample size) the sample statistics approach population parameters
  - *central limit theorem* – irrespective of the sampling distribution, as the sample size increases, the sampling distribution gets closer to a normal distribution.
  The natural history of RCT involves the following:
  - identify a research area/hypothesis
  - systematic review of literature
  - decide on the study population (sample)
  - decide on intervention
  - decide outcome measures
  - calculate the numbers required for statistical power
  - randomisation and blinding
  - data collection
  - analysis of data by intention to treat
  - reporting of the trial results – an international advisory group has come up with a standard format, called the CONSORT (CONsolidated Standards Of Reporting Trials) format, for reporting RCTs.
- *(Non-randomised) controlled clinical trial [(NR)CCT]* – this type of trial is usually

conducted in situations where randomisation is not possible, mainly due to ethical reasons. Usually a historical control is used in this type of study. Examples:
- before/after (pre-test/post-test) studies
- comparisons between matched groups
- quasi-randomised trial – in which the treatment allocation is not random.

- *Meta-analysis* – is the statistical synthesis of numerical results from several primary studies addressing the same clinical question. It is applicable only to RCTs and the aim is to produce a single precise estimate of treatment effect. It uses methods like *Mantel-Haenszel estimates* and *Peto's method* to calculate these summaries. Meta-analysis has the virtue of increasing the sample size, but has the disadvantages of heterogeneity of samples and publication bias. Meta-analysis could be carried out on the original individual data from all studies involved or on aggregated data like odds ratios from each individual study. An international advisory group has come up with a standard format, called the QUOROM (QUality Of Reporting Of Meta-analysis) statement, for reporting meta-analyses.
- *Systematic review* – is an overview of primary studies, which is conducted according to an explicit, predefined and reproducible methodology. Like any standard primary study, it contains statement of objectives, materials and methods.

The steps in conducting a systematic review are:
- formulate the question and design a rigorous methodology
- meticulous search and selection of all eligible studies
- critical appraisal of all studies
- analysing and interpreting results using appropriate statistical tests.

Systematic reviews have the following advantages:
- give precise estimates of overall treatment effects
- consistency of results across several studies helps to establish generalisability of findings and applicability to general population
- heterogeneity of results across studies gives important insights into different subgroups.

Hierarchy of evidence from research

The hierarchy of evidence from research studies is put in the following order (from best to least evidence):

1 Systematic reviews and meta-analysis.
2 RCT with definitive results (i.e. has a significant p-value and confidence interval does not include *'value of no effect'*).
3 RCT with non-definitive results (i.e. has a significant p-value but confidence interval overlaps the *'value of no effect'*).
4 Cohort studies.
5 Case control studies.
6 Cross-sectional studies.
7 Case reports.[2]

Writing a research proposal

The steps in writing a research proposal are as follows:

1 Give a short and interesting project title and mention the details of the researchers and the institution.
2 Write a brief summary of the project (like an abstract).
3 Give the background of the study and a brief literature review with appropriate references.
4 Decide the aims (the overall goals of the project) and objectives (the specific tasks in stepwise sequence which will lead to the goal) of the study, or formulate a hypothesis.
5 Briefly describe the methods to be used, including design of the study, ethical considerations, data collection and analysis, interpretation of results and report writing.
6 Describe the project milestones and devise a timetable to enable you to check that all stages will be covered and time allowed for writing up. In general, research time can be divided into thirds: one-third for planning and getting ready, one-third for data collection and one-third for analysis and writing up.
7 Describe generalisability (applicability to general population as a whole), benefits to NHS and implementation of research findings.
8 Describe the likely costing for the project and possible source of funding.
9 Apply for funding, if required.
10 Give references – use a small number of references (fewer than ten), which should be accurate and well set out, listing them in one of the standard styles, i.e. *Harvard* or *Vancouver*. The latter is the most popular style and involves numbering the references in the text, either in parentheses or superscripts, in the order in which they appear in the text. In Harvard style the name of the first author with the year of publication is cited in the text in parentheses and the reference list is written in alphabetical order.[3,6]

Organising a drug trial

The steps in organising a drug trial are as follows:

- *Identify the need for a trial and arrange necessary funding* – usually you have to find a drug company to sponsor the trial.
- *Decide on the type of study design* – whether it is retrospective or prospective; randomised or non-randomised; open/single blind or double blind; parallel group or crossover trial and placebo or conventional drug vs new drug, etc.
- *Decide on inclusion and exclusion criteria* – which are usually based on age, sex, racial and social factors and presence or absence of particular exposure, co-morbid conditions or concomitant use of other drugs, etc.
- *Define the end points (primary and secondary)* – usually mortality or development of the disease in question or development of significant side effects, etc.
- *Calculation of the power of the study* – it is important to include enough patients to enable the trial to reach statistical significance and this is usually done with the help of a statistician.
- *Ethics committee approval* – any trial should be approved by the ethics

committee as per guidelines produced by the Helsinki Convention. The ethics committee requires detailed information as to the design of the trial and a consent form needs to be approved by them.

- *Decide on statistical tools for analysis* – decide whether you need parametric or non-parametric statistical tests. The best approach is 'intention to treat analysis'.
- *Interim analysis* – it is important to analyse the end points as the trial proceeds, to detect any statistical difference should it become obvious at an early stage. Many trials have been stopped midway because a significant benefit or complication was so obvious that to continue the trial would have been unethical.[5]

Making bids and grant applications

You may have a good idea for a research project, but to pursue it you need time, materials, support and necessary finance. Making bids and grant applications is a very common thing you have to do while planning to submit your research proposal. Before embarking on your funding application, you must ask yourself the following questions:

- What is the nature of your research?
- Who funds the researchers in your area?
- Who would potentially fund your project?

To answer these questions, your first point of contact should be the research office in your college, university or hospital. The research administrator can advise you on appropriate available schemes and potential funding bodies in that field of research. He/she can also offer you guidance on the rules and regulations of the various potential funding bodies and support with the development of costings. However, you can get most of this information from your supervisor or colleagues who have gone through this process and also from various websites (e.g. www.neh.gov/grants/, www.findingagents.com).

You must start your grant research well in advance, as it is time consuming. Draw up a list of potential sponsors, search their websites to know their aims and objectives and eligibility criteria. Download appropriate forms and necessary information. You may get some of these forms from your college or university research office.

Most funding bodies have their own grant application forms and these forms should be filled up with necessary details by the applicants. Even though the details in these forms vary from sponsor to sponsor, they usually include the following points:

- *A covering letter* – to introduce yourself, your institution and the research you are doing.
- *Statement of intent* – should clearly state the following:
  - What are the main aims and objectives of your study?
  - Why is your project important and how is it different to other similar projects?
  - How is the project going to help you?
  - How will the funding body benefit from the study?
- *Research proposal* – you have to write the details of your project, as mentioned earlier under 'Writing a research proposal'.

- *Budget proposal* – this should be done very carefully. If your proposal is over-costed it will not represent value for money in the assessors' eyes and if under-costed, you may not have enough money to run the project. A high level of detail in the budget breakdown will help to reassure the assessors that the project is well thought through. You must cost everything and then check against the guidelines for what you can include in your bid. Costs in the project are calculated under the following categories:
  - establishment costs – include costs for buying new equipments, hiring a lab or renting a house, etc.
  - consumable costs – include costs for buying papers, files, ink, reagents, cabinets and postage, etc.
  - overhead costs – include the administrative and maintenance costs, which includes staffing costs.

Some funding bodies, especially commercial bodies, may need price quotes and some of them want referees. You may, sometimes, need to complete and submit a research ethics approval form along with your grant application.[6,7]

References

1   Smith R (1992) Audit and research. *BMJ.* **305**: 905–6.
2   Greenhalgh T (2001) *How to Read a Paper: The basics of evidence based medicine* (2e). BMJ Books, London.
3   Carter Y and Thomas C (eds) (1997) *Research Methods in Primary Care* (1e). Radcliffe Medical Press, Oxford and New York.
4   Pereira-Maxwell F (1998) *A–Z of Medical Statistics: a companion for critical appraisal.* Arnold, London.
5   Altman DG (1991) *Practical Statistics for Medical Research.* Chapman and Hall/CRC, London.
6   Agha R (2005) *Making Sense of Your Medical Career: your strategic guide to success* (1e). Hodder Arnold, London.
7   Reece D (ed.) (1995) *How to Do It* (3e). BMJ Publishing Group, London.

Chapter 15

Medical publications

Introduction

Before embarking on the expedition of research and publication, however small it is, you must think about it carefully and never take it lightly. The important points to consider prior to starting your new venture are:

- *Is there any compelling need to do it?* It is really hard work.
- *Do you have enough time?* It is time consuming. The time needed for your study can be divided into three equal parts – time for planning of the study and getting ready, time for collecting data, and finally time for analysing data and writing up the paper.
- *Have you got a predictable lifestyle?* You will need a stable personal, social and professional life and financial security to carry on.
- *Do you have good library facilities?* You will need them for your study.[1]

Types of publications

The common types of publications/presentations we embark on as junior doctors are as follows:

- writing a letter to a medical journal
- writing a case report
- writing an abstract
- writing a poster presentation
- writing an original article/paper
- writing a review article
- writing a book review
- writing a handbook.

How to write a paper

Objectives of publishing a paper

- Assessment of your observations by others.
- Repeat the experiment if others wish.
- To fulfil the requirement of academic career progression.

Basic structure of a paper

The basic structure of a paper conventionally follows a format known as '*IMRAD*', which is the abbreviation of Introduction, Methods, Results and Discussion. Nowadays, most journals print an *abstract* at the beginning of the paper and this is often the only part of the paper that people read. Each section of an article is meant for answering a particular question.

- *Abstract* – What is, in brief, the main message from your study?
- *Introduction* – Why did you start?
- *Methods* – What did you do?
- *Results* – What did you find?
- *Discussion* – What does it mean?

The *abstract* is a very brief and clear summary of your study and it must contain the main points that you wish to get across. An abstract must be capable of being read independently of the full report, i.e. it must stand alone. Ideally the abstract should be written after finishing writing up the article/dissertation. Every effort and sufficient time must be devoted to composing a good abstract. It should be presented exactly in the same format of 'IMRAD' as in the full article. The length of an abstract should be less than 10% of the full paper and should not exceed 250 words. When only the abstract is sent for publication or to a conference organiser, it must include the title of the article and names of authors; however, an abstract should not normally contain references. Increasingly journals are now printing structured abstracts consisting of:

- objectives
- design
- setting
- subjects
- interventions
- outcome measures
- results and
- conclusion.

The *introduction* should be brief and must state clearly the question that you tried to answer in your study. To lead the reader to this point it may be necessary to review the relevant literature briefly.

Methods – the main purpose of this section is to describe and sometimes descend the experimental design and to provide sufficient detail so that a competent worker can repeat the study.

Results – two key features of this section are:

- overall description of the major findings of the study and
- presentation of the data clearly and concisely.

Discussion – the total extent of discussion should not be more than one-third of the entire article. It should include the following points:

- summarise major findings
- discuss possible problems with the method used
- compare your results with previous works
- discuss the clinical and scientific implications of your findings
- suggest a further work
- present a succinct conclusion.

Final considerations

Once you have finished writing up your paper and the list of relevant *references* following one of the standard styles, you have to consider a few important issues before sending it for publication.

- *Try to be your own sub-editor* – you have to read your paper again and again to find out any mistakes, discrepancies, spelling and grammatical errors and make sure that the tables tally with your text.
- *Choose a better word* – you should always be in search for a better and more appropriate word in the relevant context.
- *Try to give it a short and catchy title.*
- *Find a particular journal* – which might accept your paper for publication.
- *You may have to change the style and format of your writing* – according to the requirement of a particular journal.
- *If you have to send any photograph or radiology film* – do not forget to label them on the back with authors' name, short title and indicate the 'top' with an arrow.[1,2]

How to write a letter to a medical journal

Writing a letter to a medical journal is a great way of starting your expedition for publications, as it is less stressful, less time consuming and there is a good chance of being successful by following a few simple rules.

Finding the matter for the letter

- Keep on reading different articles, editorials and case reports in the journals with a critical eye on them.
- Ask yourself:
  - Have the authors missed anything?
  - Have they made any wrong statements, or a statement not backed up by references?
  - Have they used the wrong methods, or interpreted the results wrongly?
  - Have they been carried away with their conclusions?
- If you get a positive answer to any of the above questions, then you have your material for a letter.

Writing the letter

- Start writing the letter as soon after the publication as possible.
- Get to the point immediately after 'Dear Editor'.
- Keep it short; most journals publish letters usually up to 400 words.
- Strictly follow the instructions for authors by that particular journal.
- Do not get personal; simply say why you disagree with the author.
- Support your statements with relevant references.
- Do not worry about offending the authors, but make sure that the points you are raising are important and relevant to the readers of the journal.

- Give a good title for your letter.

Do not give up if you are unsuccessful first time; put pen to paper and start again.[3]

How to write a poster presentation

Posters are not a form of publication of record, but are an important international method of communication. Nowadays, for a number of reasons, the majority of presentations at national or international scientific meetings are poster presentations.

Poster presentation is much less intimidating than oral presentation. It can allow research findings to be aired at an early stage. Presenting posters at an important meeting boosts your CV. However, producing a good poster is not an easy job. It is a creative experience, which needs good planning and hard teamworking.

Background preparations for a good poster presentation

- Viewing several posters in a national or international scientific meeting can give you an insight into the qualities of a good poster as well as some interesting ideas about selection of topics for presentations.
- Conduct a good audit study or, if possible, a research study. Write an abstract of your study and talk with your consultant about considering a poster presentation.
- Learn the art of writing a paper following the format of 'IMRAD', acknowledgement and references.
- Know the necessary software to use for preparing your poster. Microsoft PowerPoint is an ideal tool to create a poster.
- Choose the required size and orientation of your poster.
- A poster is primarily a visual presentation, so make visual impact a high priority by looking critically at the layout, using self-explanatory graphics, minimising the amount of text, using appropriate colours and leaving enough empty spaces.
- While writing a poster, keep reminding yourself that you are writing a very short story, which should have a smooth flow of clear message written with short, direct sentences and should be self-sufficient.
- Contact the medical illustration department of your hospital well in advance so that they can print your poster in time, otherwise you may have to arrange that through a private agency.

Qualities of a good poster

- Use of a single sheet of paper (ideal size A0 [120 cm × 90 cm]).
- Readable from distance of at least 1 metre.
- Colourful, with a light background.
- Good layout – ideally 20% text, 40% graphics and 40% empty space.
- Heading – the title should be large, prominent, to the point and span across

the width of the poster. The author's name should be in large type and there should be your institutional logo.
- The central question of the study stated clearly in introduction.
- Use of simple font and appropriate size of letters (suggested ideal sizes for an A0 poster: heading – largest type (48–72 point), subheading – 38 point, text – 28 point, legend – 28 point, references – 18–22 point and acknowledgements – 14–18 point).
- Use of short sentences in plain English, in active voice with minimum use of only well-known abbreviations.
- Minimum text.
- Few tables and graphics.
- Simple statistics.
- Easy to understand.
- An explicit take-home message.
- Few relevant references (≤ 5).[4–6]

How to write a good book review

Writing a book review is not too complicated and a good book review will be a publication to boost your CV as well.

Steps in writing a good book review

- *Introduce the subject, scope and the type of book.*
  - Identify the book by title, author and publishing information.
  - Specify the type of book and prospective readers.
  - Mention the book's theme.
  - You may have to give a bit of background information to enable the readers to place the book into a specific context.
- *Summarise the content of the book briefly.*
  - Provide an overview of the book's content and primary supporting points, including paraphrases and quotations from the book.
- *Provide your reaction to the book.*
  - Describe the book: is the book interesting, entertaining, useful or informative and why?
  - Respond to the author's opinion: what do you agree or disagree with and why?
  - Explore issues the book raises: what possibilities does the book suggest or leave out?
  - Relate your argument to other books or authors: support your argument for or against the author's opinions by bringing in other authors you agree with.
  - Relate the book to larger issues: how did the book affect you? How have your opinions about the topic been changed by the book?
- *Conclude by summarising your ideas.*
  - Briefly restate your main points raised in the review and close with a direct comment on the book. You may like to offer advice for potential readers.[1]

How to read a paper

Introduction

How to read a paper depends mainly on two important issues:

- 'Why do you want to read the paper?' i.e. the *purpose of your reading*.
- 'Why was the study done or what clinical question did the study try to answer?' i.e. the *purpose of the paper*.

Depending on the purpose, the reading can be classified into three types or levels as follows:

- *Browsing* – means flicking through the books or journals looking for anything that might interest us.
- *Reading for information* – in which we look through literature to find an answer to a specific question or problem.
- *Reading for research* – in which we have to go through the methodological details of the study and try to get a comprehensive view of the existing state of knowledge, ignorance and uncertainty in that particular field.

When we flick through a journal or read a journal article for some particular information, we are usually guided by the following surrounding issues:

- Is it a standard established journal?
- Is the article interesting and relevant to our practice (i.e. is it addressing an important question)?
- Is the paper published from an institution having a proven academic record?
- Are the author/s well known in that relevant field?
- Is there a good abstract of the paper?
- Is there any editorial or feedback on the paper?
- What are the dates of acceptance and publication of the paper?

Generally we do not bother too much about the methodological quality of the study. However, if we have to decide whether a paper is worth reading, we must do that on the design of the methods section only, not anything else. This is because, even if everything mentioned above sounds good, but the study design is not appropriate, then it will not give us any reliable answer to the question asked in the study. The assessment of methodological quality of a paper is known as *critical appraisal*.

Critical evaluation of a paper includes assessment of: the appropriateness of the study, the methodological nitty-gritty, statistical significance, validity of the data presented, practical implications and cost-effectiveness. To enable us to get to this point we have to have a basic understanding of various *research study designs* and necessary *medical statistics*, which have been and are discussed in the preceding and following chapters respectively. However, I am discussing briefly the necessary components of critical appraisal of a paper below.

Critical appraisal of a paper

Critical appraisal is defined as the interpretation of the strength and weakness of the research process and application of judgements to practice.

We have to ask a few preliminary questions to start critical evaluation of a paper:

- *Why was the study done?* (Is the clinical question clearly mentioned?)
- *What type of study was done?*
- *Was the study design appropriate to the broad field of research addressed?*
- *Was the study ethical?*

Further evaluation of the paper depends to some extent on what broad field of research and type of study have been addressed. However, most of the following questions are relevant to all broad fields of research and study types.

- *Was the study original?*
  (If not, did it use a more rigorous methodology/was this a larger study/was the follow-up longer than the previous similar studies, so that it can add significantly to meta-analysis of previous studies?)
- *Who is the study about?*
  (Has the study clearly mentioned the group of subjects studied, process of patients' recruitment, inclusion and exclusion criteria and whether the study was conducted in a real-life situation?)
- *Was the study design sensible?*
  (Has it clearly mentioned the specific interventions being considered, what primary and secondary outcomes were measured and how were they measured?)
- *Was the study adequately controlled?*
  (Whether the study groups were comparable; if not, whether the baseline differences have been adjusted and whether proper randomisation and blinding was done to avoid or minimise systematic bias?)
- *Was the study large enough and with long enough follow-up to make results credible?*
  (Whether the sample size was adequate and the duration and completeness of follow up were appropriate?)
- *Have the data been analysed as per the original study protocol?*
- *Were analyses performed on an intention to treatment basis?*
- *Were the statistical tests appropriate for the type of data analysed?*
- *Were appropriate measures of effect used?*
- *Have p-values and confidence intervals been calculated and interpreted appropriately?*
- *How large was the treatment effect?*
- *How precise was the estimate of treatment effect?*
- *Are the likely treatment benefits worth the potential harm or costs?*
- *Have the results been expressed in terms of risk/benefit that can be expected by an individual patient?*
- *Have the authors commented on any methodological flaws and the clinical and scientific implications of the findings of the study?*
- *Are the conclusions of the paper justified?*
- *Can the results be generalised to other populations?*
- *What is the overall impact of the paper?*

For detailed discussion on critical appraisal of papers from different types of studies, the reader is referred to Trisha Greenhalgh's *How to Read a Paper*.[7]

References

1 Reece D (ed.) (1995) *How to Do It* (3e). BMJ Publishing Group, London.
2 Hall GM (ed.) (1998) *How to Write a Paper* (2e). BMJ Books, London.
3 Walsh K (Clinical Editor, BMJ Learning) (2005) Tips on … writing a letter to a medical journal. *BMJ Careers.* 15 October. **331**: 169.
4 Durai R and Venkatraman R (2005) How to prepare a good poster. *Hospital Doctor.* 19 May.
5 Leach JP (1998) The poster session. *BMJ.* **316**: 157.
6 Kirby R and Mundy T (2002) *Succeeding as a Hospital Doctor: the experts share their secrets* (2e). Health Press, Oxford.
7 Greenhalgh T (2001) *How to Read a Paper: the basics of evidence based medicine* (2e). BMJ Books, London.

Section 5: Medical statistics

- Basics of statistics
- Descriptive statistics
- Inferential statistics
- Significance test and others
- Diagnostic statistics

Chapter 16

Basics of statistics

What are statistics?

Statistics are a collection of procedures for describing and analysing data, whereas the *data* are the numbers we get when we measure and count things in a particular context. Statistics are therefore the science of learning from data.

Types of statistics

Statistics are of two types as follows:

- *Descriptive statistics* – used to describe the characteristics of a sample and include the following:
  - methods for organising sample data
  - methods for calculating average values
  - methods for calculating values of spread
  - methods of measuring association.

  Measures of average, measures of spread and measures of association of the sample values are collectively known as *summary measures.*
- *Inferential statistics* – used to draw conclusions from a sample about the wider population from which the sample is drawn while taking into account the possible chance effects. They include the following:
  - probability theory
  - hypothesis testing
  - confidence interval analysis.

Individuals and variables

Individuals are the subjects or objects described by a set of data and *variables* are the characteristics of an individual. A variable can take different values or attributes for different individuals.

Examples of variables are age, sex, weight, height, blood groups, blood pressure, number of hospital admissions, etc.

Types of variables

There are two main types of variables as follows.

- **Categorical/qualitative variables** – these are not usually real numbers, rather they express a quality and we cannot apply rules of arithmetic to them. These variables are of two types:

– *nominal variables* – include simple names or categories and do not have any inherent orderings. Examples are yes/no, male/female, dead/alive, blood groups O/A/B/AB, etc.

– *ordinal variables* – the variables used to describe grades or stages and they have a natural or inherent ordering or ranking. Examples are grades or stages of a disease, degree of satisfaction (satisfied/undecided/unsatisfied), classes of heart failure or chest pain, level of improvement (much better/better/same/worse) or agreement (strongly agree/agree/neutral/disagree/strongly disagree), etc.

• **Metric/numerical/quantitative variables** – have precisely defined values and are real numbers which can be counted or measured. We can apply all rules of arithmetic to these data. These variables are of two types:

– *continuous variables* – can take an unlimited number of values within a given range and the data usually come from *measuring* things. Examples are temperature, height, weight, volume, pressure, etc., all of which are metric variables

– *discrete variables* – can take a limited number of values or categories and the data usually come from *counting* things. Examples are number of children per couple, number of births/deaths/hospital admissions, etc. (All nominal and ordinal variables are discrete variables as well.)

Discrete variables which can take only two values (e.g. yes/no, male/female, married/unmarried, etc.) are known as *dichotomous variables* and the data are called *binary data*.

Some uncommon types of data

• *Ranks, scores, visual analogue scales, etc.* – this type of data should be handled cautiously. Analysis should be carried out using a rank-based method rather than their exact values.

• *Censored data* – the data we get when we cannot measure the value of a variable precisely but we know that it is beyond some limit. For example:

– In laboratory testing when we measure some trace constituents of blood (e.g. TSH – thyroid-stimulating hormone), the actual level may be below the lowest possible level the machine can detect and this lowest possible detectable level is obviously not zero. These values lower than the level of detectability are termed non-detectable. We report the result as < the limit of detectability, which is a censored value at this limit. As conventionally we plot data with lower values to the left on a horizontal scale, it is known as *left censoring*.

– In survival studies, there is usually a fixed length of follow-up period and so the *outcome of interest* (death, appearance or disappearance of a disease, etc.) will not happen to every individual of the study at the end of that period. Therefore, at the end of follow-up many individuals will still be alive and we do not know how long they will survive. We can only say that their survival time will be longer than the period of follow-up (i.e. > the arbitrary fixed length of follow-up). This survival time is called *censored*, to indicate that the period of observation was cut off before the outcome of interest occurred. As the values are greater than the limit, it is also known as *right censoring*.

- Withdrawals from trials at different points of time before the end of the follow-up period also lead to censored observations and data.

Populations and samples

A *population* in statistics means a complete collection of a defined group of *individuals* (people, objects or items) in which we have an interest. Examples are all schoolchildren in England, all drug addicts in London, all patients with stroke in a particular area, all prescriptions written from a GP surgery over a month, etc.

A population includes every eligible member of the group however defined. Due to a number of reasons (e.g. too large or too volatile population, limited resources, ethical and safety issues, etc.), study of the whole population is impractical in most cases. To resolve this practical problem we draw a relatively small number of members from the population which is presumed to be a true representative of that population, i.e. that all the features of the population are accurately reflected in this small group called a *sample*.

The measures of characteristics of a sample (like mean, median or standard deviation) are known as *statistics* and usually expressed by English letters (e.g. x = mean, SD = standard deviation), whereas the corresponding characteristics in the population are called *parameters* and usually expressed by Greek letters (e.g. μ (mu) = mean, σ (sigma) = standard deviation).

Increasing the sample size follows the following basic statistical concepts:

- *Law of large numbers* – when we draw independent observations from a population, as the number of observations increases, the sample statistics eventually approach the population parameters.
- *Central limit theorem* – irrespective of the sampling distribution (if not a normal distribution), as the sample size increases, the sampling distribution gets closer to a normal distribution.

Measures of effect

Measures of effect are the measures used to compare differences between two or more comparison groups. There are different measures of effect in different types of data. The most common measures of effect for continuous (quantitative) data are *mean* and *median*; whereas *relative risk* and *odds ratio* are the most common measures of effect for categorical data.[1,2]

References

1   Altman DG (1991) *Practical Statistics for Medical Research*. Chapman and Hall/CRC, London.
2   Bowers D (2002) *Statistics From Scratch: an introduction for health care professionals* (2e). Wiley, Chichester.

Chapter 17

Descriptive statistics

Organising data

After collecting the raw data, they are screened and listed into a number of categories with their respective frequencies in a table. A simple way to order and display data is to use a *stem and leaf plot*, which suits small data sets.

Frequency distribution

A frequency distribution is a list of categories that a variable can take together with a count of the number of items in each category. When there are only a few categories (usually up to 15) they could be listed with one row for each category and this is called an ungrouped distribution. However, when there are many different categories they are grouped into a smaller and manageable number of classes for better understanding and analysis, which is called a grouped distribution.

Charting data

Displaying data in the form of a chart often provides us with a more immediate impressionistic view and further insights into features and patterns in the data. There are a number of charts available for displaying different types of data as follows.

Charts for qualitative data

- Bar charts.
- Pie charts.
- Line charts.
- Step charts (for cumulative frequency).

Bar charts

Bar charts are best used to display qualitative data with a small number of categories and more than one variable can be plotted in the same chart. The bars are all of the same width, equally spaced and the height of each bar represents the frequency of the corresponding category. For example, the distribution of patients with a particular diagnosis among seven consultants can be plotted as in Figure 17.1.

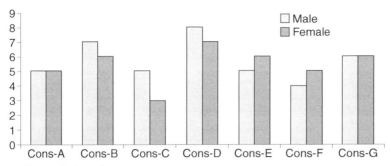

Figure 17.1 Example bar chart.

Pie charts

A pie chart is an alternative to a bar chart, but it can display only one variable. The angle of each slice of the pie is proportional to the frequency of the corresponding category and it is expressed in percentages. For example, the distribution of 50 consecutive asthma patients according to severity (mild, moderate or severe) can be displayed as shown in Figure 17.2.

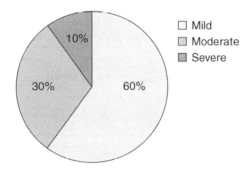

Figure 17.2 Example pie chart.

Line charts

Line charts are used to display data with a chronological basis, i.e. the data consist of regular measurements over a time period, which is known as longitudinal data. For example, the number of daily admissions in a medical admission unit over a week can be plotted as shown in Figure 17.3.

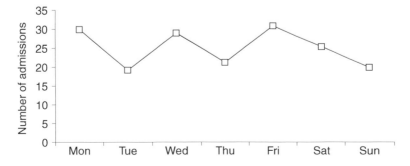

Figure 17.3 Example line chart.

Charts for discrete quantitative data

- Dot plots.
- Scatter plots.
- Frequency diagrams.
- Step charts (for cumulative frequency).

Dot plots and scatter plots

Dot plots and scatter plots are used to display ungrouped discrete data. For example, the relation between age and height in 20 children can be displayed in a scatter plot as shown in Figure 17.4.

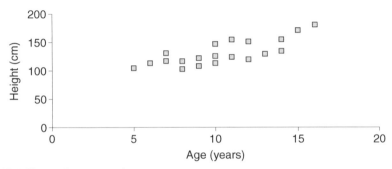

Figure 17.4 Example scatter plot.

Charts for continuous quantitative data

- Frequency histograms.
- Frequency polygons.
- Frequency curves.
- Box-whisker plots.

Frequency histograms

Histograms are used to display continuous grouped frequency distributions. If the widths of the columns are the same, the height of each column is equal to the

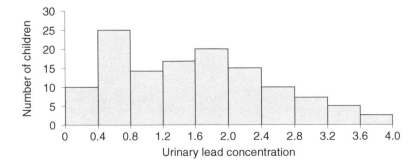

Figure 17.5 Example histogram.

corresponding class frequency. There is no gap between the bars/columns, which reflects the continuous nature of the data. Urinary lead concentration in a group of urban children is displayed in the histogram in Figure 17.5.

Frequency polygons

If we connect the midpoints of all the columns of a histogram then we will get a curve, which is called a frequency polygon. A smooth frequency polygon is known as a frequency curve.

Frequency curves

The inherent patterns in the sample data are best understood by constructing charts. However, if the data are so distributed that we can draw a smooth curve through a frequency histogram or polygon then we get the ultimate realisation of this pattern and this curve is called a *frequency curve*. A frequency curve may be symmetrical or asymmetrical.

Normal distribution

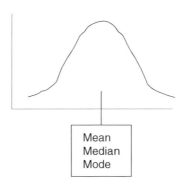

Negatively skewed   **Positively skewed**

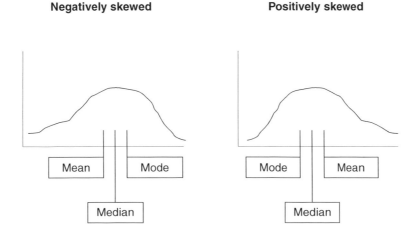

Figure 17.6 Example frequency curves.

A frequency distribution which has a smooth symmetric bell-shaped curve that can be described by a mathematical equation is known as *normal distribution*.

An asymmetrical frequency curve having a longer tail on one side than the other indicates a *skewed distribution*. When the frequency curve has a longer tail on the right side it is called *right or positively skewed* and similarly if the left tail is longer it is known as *left or negatively skewed* (*see* Figure 17.6).

A frequency curve which is flatter than normal distribution is called a *platokurtic* curve and one peakier than normal distribution is known as a *leptokurtic* curve.

Box-whisker plots

A box-whisker plot is a graph of five-number summary and is used to display a large data set. The bottom and top of the box mark the first and third quartiles (Q1 and Q3) and the interval between these two is known as the interquartile range (IQR). The horizontal line in the middle of the box marks the median and the ends of the whiskers indicate the smallest and the largest sample values (i.e. the range). (*See* Figure 17.7.)

Boxplots can be used for side-by-side comparison of more than one distribution. Any observation lying 1.5 × IQR above Q3 or below Q1 is called a suspected *outlier*.

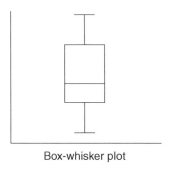

Box-whisker plot

Figure 17.7 Example box-whisker plot.

Probability distribution of data

Many statistical methods are based on the assumption that the observed sample data are from a population with a particular theoretical distribution. This distributional assumption helps us to decide whether to analyse the data using *parametric* or *non-parametric methods* (discussed later). A few common probability distributions are as follows:

- *Normal distribution* – by far the most important probability distribution in medical research, as many biological parameters follow normal distribution in the population. This is also known as *Gaussian* distribution, after the German mathematician CF Gauss (1777–1855). It is unimodal and symmetrical. The most important characteristic of normal distribution is that it is completely described by two parameters – *mean* and *standard deviation*.
- *Lognormal distribution* – taking logarithms of data with some skewed distribution

often gives a near-normal distribution. After gaining near-normality by taking logs of original data, we perform the statistical tests and finally we take the antilog of the derived data (e.g. mean and standard deviation) to get the ultimate result.

- *Binominal distribution* – this is the simplest probability distribution for binary data, i.e. discrete data with only two probabilities. The distribution is asymmetrical, but with increased sample size it becomes more symmetrical like normal distribution.
- *Poisson distribution* – named after the French mathematician SD Poisson (1781–1840), and is a specific distribution of discrete data, which arises when we count the number of occurrences of an event over time or on different subjects. The distribution is asymmetrical, but with increasing sample size, like binominal distribution, this distribution looks like normal distribution.[1-3]

Measures of average or location

The commonly used measures are as follows.

- *Mean* – the conventional average, which is calculated by adding up all the sample values and then dividing by the number of values:

$$\therefore x = \Sigma\, X/n$$

where 'x' = mean; 'Σ' (Greek capital sigma) = sum of/summation; 'X' = each of the sample values; 'n' = total number of sample values.
- *Median* – the middle or central value after the sample values have been arranged in ascending order. If the sample values are even in number then the median is the average of the middle two values.
- *Mode* – the value that occurs most frequently in the sample data and measures the most typical value. A sample data having two modes is known to have a *bimodal distribution*.
- *Percentiles* – the values which identify or locate any specified percentage of the whole sample. For example, the values below which 10% or 25% of the sample values lie are known as 10th or 25th percentile respectively. The *50th percentile* divides the sample values into two equal halves and represents the *median* of the sample. The *25th, 50th* and *75th* percentiles are of particular interest as they divide the frequency distribution of the sample values into four equal parts and are known as first, second and third *quartiles*. The interval between the first and third quartiles is called interquartile range (IQR). IQR represents the mid 50% of the distribution and is an important measure of location, especially in skewed distribution.

For metric data we can choose any of the measures of average from mean, median or mode and the choice depends mainly on which aspect of the average we wish to capture. For ordinal data mean should not be used and so the choice remains between median and mode. However, for nominal data the only suitable measure of average is mode. As a rule of the thumb the most appropriate measures of average are:

- *mean* for metric data

- *median* for ordinal and skewed metric data
- *mode* for nominal data.

If the frequency distribution is symmetrical then all three measures will be identical. If the frequency distribution is right or positively skewed then *mean > median > mode*; whereas in a left or negatively skewed distribution *mean < median < mode*.[2]

Measures of spread or dispersion

Measures of spread or dispersion basically means the average distance of the sample values from the central value of the distribution. There are three types of spread measures:

- **Frequency-based measures** – are based on the way in which the sample values are spread out among different categories or classes. They are principally used with nominal and non-numeric ordinal variables and include the *variation ratio (VR)*, *index of diversity (ID)* and *index of qualitative variation (IQV)*.
- **Range-based measures** – are based on the difference between the largest and the smallest values in the sample. They are used mainly with the numeric ordinal and skewed metric variables and include the *range, interquartile range (IQR)* and *semi-interquartile range (SIQR)*.
- **Deviation-based measures** – are based on the average difference or deviation between each sample value and the mean of the sample values. These are used with quantitative variables and include the most important measure of spread for quantitative variables – the *standard deviation (SD)*.

Unlike the range, the standard deviation uses every data point and gives us a more precise idea about the distribution of the data in the sample. A large SD means there is a lot of variation from the mean, whereas a small SD means few data are different from the mean. The combination of mean and standard deviation for normally distributed data is a very powerful tool, because they can be analysed by most parametric tests.

Steps in calculating standard deviation

Step 1: Calculate the sample mean value (x).

Step 2: Subtract this mean value from each observation (X) to get the *mean deviation* values: $(X - x)$.

Step 3: Square each of these mean deviation values: $(X - x)^2$.

Step 4: Add these squared values together: $\{\Sigma(X - x)^2\}$.

Step 5: Divide the sum by $(n-1)$, i.e. the degree of freedom. The result is known as *variance*: $\{\Sigma(X - x)^2/(n - 1)\}$.

Step 6: Take the square-root of the variance and the result is the *standard deviation*:

$$SD = \sqrt{\{\Sigma(X - x)^2/(n - 1)\}}$$

When the sample values have a normal frequency distribution, *68%* (68.27%) of sample values will lie within *one SD* of the mean and the corresponding figures within *two* and *three SD* of the mean are *95.45%* (95% within *1.96 SD*) and *99.73%* (99% within *2.58 SD*).[2] (*See* Figure 17.8.)

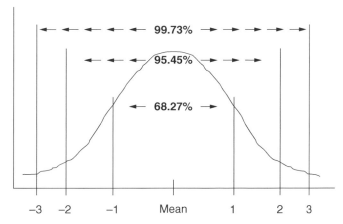

Figure 17.8 Standard deviation and Normal frequency distribution.

Measures of association

Correlation and regression

Correlation and regression are the techniques for dealing with the relationship or associations between two or more *continuous variables*. (Chi-square (χ^2) statistics are used for examining associations between *categorical variables*.)

Although these two terms are often presented together, they are different methods and serve distinct purposes.

Correlation

Correlation denotes association between two quantitative variables. The direction and strength of association are measured by a *correlation coefficient (r)*, which takes values between (+) 1 and (–) 1. Complete absence of correlation is represented by 0, whereas complete or perfect correlation between two variables is expressed either by (+) 1 or (–) 1. A *positive correlation* is one in which both variables increase together. A *negative correlation* is one in which one variable decreases as the other increases.

If change in one variable depends on change in another variable or the intention is to make inferences about one variable from the other, then the first variable is known as the *dependent (response/outcome) variable* and the other as the *independent (predictor/explanatory) variable*. In graphical representation the dependent variable is usually plotted along the vertical axis or *y-axis* and the independent variable along the base line or *x-axis*.

For example: Figure 17.9a, a scatter plot showing the association between age and height of a group of children, reveals a positive correlation *(r = 1)*. Figure 17.9b, showing the association between age and CD4 cell count, reveals a negative correlation *(r = –1)*.

The correlation coefficient may be parametric (*Pearson's correlation coefficient*) or non-parametric (*Spearman's rank correlation coefficient*). Parametric *r* quantifies the extent of any linear increase or decrease; whereas non-parametric *r* quantifies

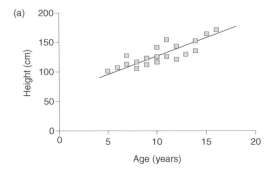

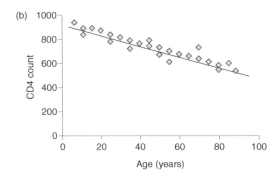

Figure 17.9a,b (a) Positive correlation; (b) Negative correlation.

the extent of any *tendency* for one variable to increase or decrease as the other increases.

The *Pearson's r* is calculated as:

$$r = \Sigma(X - x)(Y - y)/\sqrt{\{\Sigma(X - x)^2(Y - y)^2\}}$$

where 'X' represents the values of independent variable, 'Y' represents the values of the dependent variable and 'x' and 'y' denote the means of them respectively.

The *Spearman's* rank correlation coefficient (r_s) is calculated as:

$$r_s = 1 - \{6\Sigma d^2/n(n^2 - 1)\}$$

where '*d*' is the difference in ranks of the two variables for a given individual and '*n*' is the number of observations or categories.

The correlation coefficient is unaffected by the unit of measurement and it cannot be used if the relationship is not linear. Correlation may be strongly affected by a few outlying observations. A significant correlation does not imply cause and effect relationship (i.e. correlation is not causation). However, the square of the correlation coefficient (r^2) gives the proportion of the variation of one variable explained by the other.

Regression

Correlation just indicates the strength of association as a single number, but cannot predict the value of one variable from the value of the other variable and for this we need another method called *regression*. Regression estimates the dependence of the dependent variable on the independent variable and the relationship is summarised by an equation known as the *regression equation* consisting of a slope and an intercept.

The regression equation is expressed as:

$$y = \alpha + \beta x$$

where 'y' is the dependent variable, 'x' is the independent variable, 'α' is the intercept representing the value of the dependent variable when the independent variable takes the value '0', and 'β' is the slope representing the amount the dependent variable increases with unit increase in the independent variable. The slope 'β' is sometimes called the *regression coefficient*.

There are several possible approaches for regression analysis, but the most commonly used standard method is called *least square regression analysis*. This method helps to fit a regression line that minimises the distance between the data and the fitted line. Vertical measurement of the distance between the observations and the fitted line helps to minimise the sum of the squares of these distances and also it does not depend on the scaling of the graph. The value given by the fitted line for any individual observation is called *fitted value* and the technical term for the distance between the two is a *residual*.

When there are more than one independent variables, the relationship is summarised by an equation known as the *multiple regression equation* and is expressed as follows:

$$y = \alpha + \beta_1 x_1 + \beta_2 x_2 + \ldots \ldots + \beta_n x_n$$

where 'x_1' is the first independent variable, 'x_2' is the second and so on up to the 'nth' independent variable 'x_n'. However, when one of the variables is categorical (e.g. a binary outcome variable), we have to use a slightly different technique called *multiple logistic regression*.[1,4,5]

References

1   Altman DG (1991) *Practical Statistics for Medical Research*. Chapman and Hall/CRC, London.
2   Bowers D (2002) *Statistics From Scratch: an introduction for health care professionals* (2e). Wiley, Chichester.
3   Bland M (2000) *An Introduction to Medical Statistics* (3e). Oxford Medical Publications, Oxford.
4   Bowers D (1997) *Statistics Further From Scratch: for health care professionals* (1e). Wiley, Chichester.
5   Swinscow TDV and Campbell MJ (2002) *Statistics at Square One* (10e). BMJ Books, London.

Chapter 18

Inferential statistics

Probability theory

The main purpose of inferential statistics is to draw conclusions about the true but unknown population parameter from the available sample statistics. A sample is unlikely to have exactly the same features and characteristics of the original population, and so the sample statistics can never be exactly the same as the population parameter. The process of statistical inference thus has a degree of uncertainty, as we are never sure how representative of the population the sample is.

The theory of probability enables us to link samples to population, and to draw realistic conclusions about populations from samples. The following are the simple *properties of probability*:

- A probability lies between 0 (0%) and 1 (100%). A probability of 0 means that the event never happens and a probability of 1 means that the event always happens.
- The sum of the probabilities of all outcomes from an experiment must equal 1.
- *Addition rule* – when two events are *mutually exclusive*, i.e. when one happens the other cannot happen, then the probability that one or the other happens is the sum of their probabilities. For example, a rolling dice may show a one or two, but not both together. The probability that it shows a one or two = 1/6 + 1/6 = 2/6.
- *Multiplication rule* – when two events are *independent*, i.e. knowing one has happened does not affect the happening of the other, the probability that both will happen is the product of their probabilities. For example, if we toss a coin twice, the second toss will be independent of the first toss. The probability of two heads or two tails occurring is ½ × ½ = ¼.

From a statistical viewpoint there are main three approaches in *calculating the probability* of any outcome:

- *Classic (mathematical) approach* – is based on the work of early researchers in probability theory. However, this approach only works with experiments where all outcomes have an equal chance of happening (like tossing a coin or rolling a dice) and it has very little relevance in any practical biomedical experiments.
- *Frequentist approach/definition* – states that the probability of occurrence of a particular event equals the proportion of times the event occurs in a large number of repeated trials in the long run. This method depends on the existence of frequency data from identical or very similar experiments in the past. This is a much more useful method and usually used in statistics.

- *Subjective approach/definition* – depends simply on one's subjective belief in the occurrence of an event or in a hypothesis. This is the only feasible approach where suitable frequency data do not exist. This definition corresponds more closely with everyday uses and is the foundation of the Bayesian approach to statistics. This approach is quite different from the frequentist approach and not widely used nowadays. In this approach the investigator assigns a prior or pre-test probability to an event (or a hypothesis) under investigation. Then the study is carried out, the data collected and the probability is modified in the light of the results obtained. The revised probability is called posterior or post-test probability.

Bayes' theorem

Bayes' theorem was named after the English clergyman Thomas Bayes (1702–1761), who is considered the father of the principle behind this statistical approach. It explains a mathematical equation which gives the conditional probability of an event, i.e. the probability that an event will occur given that another condition is also present. This is the basis for the calculation of the probability of disease given the results of relevant diagnostic tests. It includes:

- the predictive value of a test
- the multiplication rule
- independence and mutually exclusive events.

Essentially it allows us to revise our initial hypothesis on the level of disease in the light of further diagnostic information. We start with an initial hypothesis called a *prior* or *pre-test probability.* Then we apply the test, in which we know the characteristics. Based on the test information we modify our hypothesis to give a *posterior* or *post-test probability* (*see* Figure 18.1).

- Pre-test odds = pre-test probability/(1 – pre-test probability).
- Post-test odds = pre-test odds × likelihood ratio.
- Post-test probability = post-test odds/(1 + post-test odds).

The following is an example of Bayesian analysis (if conditional independence holds).

1 A man attends A&E with a history of chest pain. What is the probability of him having a myocardial infarction (MI)?
   - The prevalence of MI in those attending A&E with chest pain is 20%.
   - Therefore the *pre-test probability* of him having an MI = *0.20.*
   - The pre-test odds = 0.20/(1 – 0.20) = 0.25.

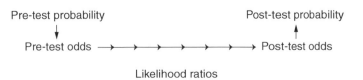

Figure 18.1 Steps in Bayesian analysis.

2 Now, we know that he is *60 years old*. How is this going to modify the probability?
   - The likelihood ratio of having an MI in a 60-year-old man with chest pain is 1.8.
   - Therefore the post-test odds = 0.25 × 1.8 = 0.45.
   - The *post-test probability* of having an MI = 0.45/(1 + 0.45) = 0.31.
3 However, if the patient says that his *chest pain radiates to his left arm*, but with *no associated sweating*, how will this modify the probability?
   - Chest pain radiating to left arm has a +ve LR for MI = 2.7.
   - Chest pain without sweating has a −ve LR for MI = 0.52.
   - Therefore the post-test odds = 0.25 × 1.8 × 2.7 × 0.52 = 0.63.
   - The *post-test probability* of having an MI = 0.63/(1 + 0.63) = *0.39*.

Thus, a 60-year-old man presenting with chest pain radiating to the left arm but without associated sweating has a *39%* probability of having an MI.[1-3]

Hypothesis testing

Null hypothesis

When an investigator conducts a study he or she usually has a theory in mind; for example, patients with diabetes have high blood pressure, or oral contraceptives may cause breast cancer. This theory is known as the *study hypothesis*. However, it is impossible to prove most hypotheses, as one can always think of circumstances, which have not yet arisen, under which the hypothesis may not hold. There is a simpler logical setting for disproving hypotheses than for proving them. The converse of the study hypothesis is known as the *null hypothesis*; e.g. diabetic patients do not have high blood pressure or oral contraceptives do not cause breast cancer. Such a hypothesis is usually phrased in the negative and that is why it is termed *null*.

Hypothesis testing is a method of deciding whether the data are consistent with the null hypothesis. When we conduct a study to compare between two groups, the null hypothesis states that there is no difference between the two group statistics. We then analyse the data to determine whether we are right or wrong. If we find a significant difference, then the null hypothesis is wrong and we *reject* it; if we do not find any significant difference, then the null hypothesis is true and we *fail to reject* it.

Type 1 error

To reject the null hypothesis when in fact it is true is to make what is known as *type 1 error*. The level at which a result is declared significant is known as the *type 1 error rate* or *α*. A type 1 error is often more serious than a type 2 error and so every effort should be made to avoid this. The hypothesis test procedure is therefore adjusted to guarantee a low probability of rejecting the null hypothesis wrongly; however, this probability is never 0. The probability of type 1 error is expressed as:

$$p \text{ (type 1 error)} = \text{significance level} = \alpha$$

The *significance level* of a statistical hypothesis test is a *fixed probability* of wrongly rejecting the null hypothesis (when it is in fact true). This significance level is set by the investigator in relation to the consequence of such an error. We want to make a significance level as small as possible in order to protect the null hypothesis and at the same time to prevent the investigator from inadvertently making false claims. Usually, the significance level is chosen at 5% or 1%, i.e. $\alpha = 0.05$ or 0.01.

Type 2 error

The failure to reject the null hypothesis when in fact it is false is known as a *type 2 error*. The *type 2 error rate* is denoted as β. A type 2 error is frequently due to too small a sample size. The exact probability of a type 2 error (β) is generally unknown, but it becomes smaller with increasing sample size.

The *power* of a statistical hypothesis test measures the test's ability to reject the null hypothesis when it is actually false, i.e. to make a correct decision. In other words, the power of a hypothesis test is the probability of not committing a type 2 error. This is calculated by subtracting the probability of a type 2 error from 1, and usually expressed as:

$$power = 1 - p \text{ (type 2 error)} = (1 - \beta)$$

The maximum power of a test can be 1, and the minimum is 0. Ideally we want a test to have high power, close to 1.

For a given set of data, type 1 and type 2 errors are inversely related, i.e. the smaller the risk of one, the higher the risk of the other, and we have to keep that in mind when setting the significance level, α. (*See* Table 18.1.)

Table 18.1 Type 1 and type 2 errors

		Null hypothesis	
		False	*True*
Test result	*Significant*	Power	Type 1 error
	Non-significant	Type 2 error	Insufficient evidence

P-value

When we are studying the difference between two groups (e.g. blood pressure in diabetic and non-diabetic patients or incidence of lung cancer in non-smokers and smokers) we must expect some difference due to *random variation* or *chance* alone. We have to set a level of significance or limits before deciding whether the null hypothesis is true or false on the basis of the study results.

The probability of obtaining an observed result in a study *by chance*, if the null hypothesis is true, is known as the *p-value*. If the *p-value* is less than the set significance level (α) of the test, i.e. $p < \alpha$ *(type 1 error rate)*, then the observed result is significant and we reject the null hypothesis.

Since the *p-value* is a probability, it takes values between 0 and 1. Values near to zero suggest that the null hypothesis is unlikely to be true. The smaller the *p-value* the more significant is the result. Conventionally we take 5% (p = 0.05) as the level of significance and we can get that by setting the limits at twice the standard error of the difference. Therefore a difference greater than the limits we have set is significant and makes the null hypothesis unlikely. However, a difference within the set limits which is regarded as non-significant does not make the null hypothesis likely, but it suggests that insufficient information is available to reject the null hypothesis. If p = 0.05 or 0.01 this means the result is significant at 5% or 1% respectively; in other words the sample difference has a 1 in 20 or 1 in 100 chance respectively of occurring if the null hypothesis is true.

Z-test and z-scores

The 'z-test' is a significance test which is used for comparing *means* or *proportions* between two groups. 'Z-scores' are measurements which are expressed in units of *standard deviation (SD)* or *standard error (SE)* and they are obtained by subtracting the mean from individual measurements (which follow a normal distribution) and dividing the result by the standard deviation *(SD)*. So:

$$z\text{-score} = (\text{observation} - \text{mean})/\text{SD}$$

For example, if the mean height of a group of people is 170 cm with SD of 10 cm, a person measuring 180 cm has a z-score of 1 (i.e. + 1 SD away from the mean).

Z-scores are used to assess the significance of a result by finding the appropriate *p-value* in relation to the z-score from the *'P-value table for normal distribution'* (*see* Appendix 1). The *higher the z-score*, the *smaller is the p-value*, i.e. the result is unlikely to occur by chance.

Steps in calculating the p-value

Step 1: Calculate the sample mean *(x)*.
Step 2: Calculate the standard deviation *(SD)* of the mean.
Step 3: Calculate the z-score: *z-score = (observed value – mean)/SD*.
Step 4: Find the p-value in relation to z-score from the *'P-value table for normal distribution'*.

For example, in a study, the mean difference in diastolic blood pressure (BP) between diabetics and non-diabetics was 6 mmHg and its standard error was 1.50 mmHg. Now, we can assess whether this difference in BP of 6 mmHg is significant or has arisen by chance, by using the z-score. Here the z-score is: 6/1.50 = 4, which means that this result is 4 SD away from the mean. From the 'P-value table' we find that an SD of 3.291 represents a p-value of 0.001. Therefore, the above study result, being 4 SD away from the mean, has a p-value of < 0.001 and is unlikely to be found by chance, i.e. the result is significant.

The *p-values* discussed so far are known as *two-sided p-values*, as the extreme results can occur by chance equally often in either direction from the mean. In most cases this is the correct procedure and most statisticians advocate their routine use. However, in rare cases, it is reasonable to consider that a real difference can occur only in one direction and it is reasonable to calculate a *one-sided p-value* by considering only one tail of the distribution of the test statistic. In normal distribution, the usual two-sided cut-off points at 10%, 5%, 1% and 0.1% are 1.645, 1.960, 2.576 and 3.291; however, the corresponding one-sided cut-off points are

1.282, 1.645, 2.325 and 3.090. The differences are not particularly large, but can lead to different interpretation at a fixed level of statistical significance.

There are a few limitations or problems with p-values as follows:

- The p-value is an *arbitrary value* ($p < 0.05/0.01/0.001$, etc.) that is chosen at random.
- It suggests a cut-off-point or *dichotomy* ($p < 0.05$ is significant but $p = 0.05$ is not significant), where in fact this probability is a continuum.
- A p-value greater than α (significance level $> 0.01/0.05$) *cannot differentiate* between true non-significance and small sample size.
- The p-value bears no resemblance to *clinical significance*.[4-6]

Confidence interval analysis

Standard error of mean (SEM or SE)

When we are studying a population we do not know the population mean (μ) or the standard deviation of the population mean (σ); we have only the mean of our sample to guide us. If we draw a series of samples from a large population and calculate the mean of the sample values in each of them, then we get a series of means. This series of means, like the series of observations in each sample, has a standard deviation. This standard deviation of the series of means is known as the *standard error of mean* of one sample. *This standard error (SE) is a measure of how precisely the sample mean approximates the population mean.* Repeated sampling from the population is a concept, but in fact we do not have to do that to calculate the standard error of the mean. It is calculated by dividing the SD by the square-root of the number of observations:

$$SEM = SD/\sqrt{n}$$

As with standard deviation, we can predict that a *sample mean* has a 95% chance of lying within its two standard error from the *population mean*; in other words, a mean that departs by more than twice its standard error from the population mean would be expected by chance only in about 5% of the samples.

The standard error of a proportion is calculated by the formula:

$$SE = \sqrt{(pq/n)}$$

where 'p' = proportion, 'q' = $(1 - p)$ and 'n' = sample size.

Confidence interval (CI)

The formal dictionary definition of *confidence interval* is:

> *a range of values for a variable of interest constructed so that this range has a specified probability of including the true value of the variable. The specified probability is called the* confidence level, *and the end points of the confidence interval are called the* confidence limits.

The CI thus defines a range of values within which our true but unknown population mean value (μ) is likely to lie, with a given level of confidence, i.e. CI is an *interval estimate* of a parameter (μ), whereas the value of sample mean (x) is only a *point estimate* of the population mean (μ) and is likely to be inaccurate.

Conventionally we take 95% as the level of statistical significance and so it is called *95% confidence interval (95% CI)*. As the sample mean has a 95% chance to lie within its two standard error from the population mean, we can define *95% CI = $\mu \pm 1.96$ SE*. However, we do not know the true value of μ. The best available data in hand about our population is the sample mean, x. Conventionally, the best possible estimate of the confidence interval is measured using this sample mean. And so, *95% CI = $x \pm 1.96$ SE*. Similarly we can calculate *90% CI = $x \pm 1.64$ SE* and *99% CI = $x \pm 2.58$ SE*. The narrower the range, the more accurate is the estimate.

The confidence limits, i.e. the upper and lower bounds of the interval, give us information on how big or small the true effect might plausibly be, whereas the interval estimate, i.e. the width of the confidence interval, conveys some other useful information. If the confidence interval is narrow, it indicates that the estimate of true effect is quite precise and the study has reasonable power (usually quite a large study) to detect an effect. If the confidence interval is quite wide, it suggests that the estimate of effect size is quite imprecise and it is a low-powered study (probably quite small).

Standard error (SE) and confidence interval (CI) analysis can be done on a number of parameters like *means, proportions, difference between means or proportions, regression coefficients, correlation coefficients and relative risks.*

In case of means, the formula (*95% CI = $x \pm 1.96 \times$ SE*) applies for large samples. For smaller samples (roughly < 30), to get a reliable and accurate result, the SE of the estimate should be multiplied by the critical value of t, which can be found in the tables of the t-distribution against the appropriate number of degrees of freedom (the t-test).

If the measure of effect is a *difference* (e.g. mean or absolute risk reduction), the confidence interval should not include *zero (0)*, as this means that there is no difference between the comparing groups. Similarly, when the measure of effect is a *ratio* (e.g. relative risk, risk ratio, rate ratio, odds ratio or hazard ratio), the confidence interval should not include *one (1)*, as this means no difference between the groups. Thus, '0' in case of difference and '1' in case of ratio are known as *'values of no difference or effect'*.

The confidence interval gives us two important pieces of information:

- *Statistical significance* – if the CI embraces the value of no difference, then the findings are non-significant, whereas the findings are statistically significant if the confidence interval does not include the value of no difference. Thus the CI provides us with the same information as the p-value.
- *Clinical significance* – the confidence limits tell us how large or small the real effect might be and yet still give us the observed findings by chance. This information is very helpful in interpreting both borderline significance and non-significance. Thus, CI is superior to the p-value, as it gives us the range of possible effect sizes.

However, CI has some *limitations*:

- Even very large samples and very narrow confidence intervals can be misleading if they come from biased studies, so bias must be assessed before CI can be interpreted.

- Statistical non-significance implied by CI does not mean 'no effect'. Small studies often report non-significance even when there are important, real effects.
- Statistical significance implied by CI does not necessarily mean that the effect is real. With 95% CI, there is a 1 in 20 chance of finding a significant result by chance alone.
- Statistical significance does not necessarily mean clinically important. It is the size of the effect that determines the importance, not the presence of statistical significance. For example, in a drug trial it was found that the drug raised systolic blood pressure by 1 mmHg, which was statistically significant, but this is very unlikely to be clinically significant.
- Neither the confidence intervals nor the p-values help us to decide whether significant findings from a particular study will be applicable to other groups of patients. This *external validity* of the trial findings should be based on the patients' characteristics, the setting and the conduct of the trial.

Steps in calculating confidence intervals

Step 1: Calculate the sample mean *(x)*.
Step 2: Calculate the sample standard deviation *(SD)*.
Step 3: Calculate the standard error of mean *(SE)*: *(SE = SD/√n)*.
Step 4: Choose the *desired level of confidence* and corresponding *z-score* (90% = 1.64, 95% = 1.96, or 99% = 2.58).
Step 5: Multiply *z*-score by standard error *(z × SE)*.
Step 6: Confidence interval = *x* ± *(z × SE)*.[2,4,6,7]

The steps in calculating mean, standard deviation, p-value and confidence interval in the above discussion and also the steps in performing *t*-test and χ^2-test, discussed in the appendices, are only for better understanding these issues; in fact we never have to do these manually and practically it is impossible except in the case of a very small sample. All these calculations are done by the computer using one of the statistical software packages, e.g. SPSS (Statistical Package for the Social Sciences).[2,8,9]

References

1 Bland M (2000) *An Introduction to Medical Statistics* (3e). Oxford Medical Publications, Oxford.
2 Bowers D (1997) *Statistics Further From Scratch: for health care professionals* (1e). Wiley, Chichester.
3 Kirkwood BR and Sterne J (2003) *Essential Medical Statistics* (2e). Blackwell Science, Oxford.
4 Altman DG (1991) *Practical Statistics for Medical Research.* Chapman and Hall/CRC, London.
5 Pereira-Maxwell F (1998) *A–Z of Medical Statistics: a companion for critical appraisal.* Arnold, London.
6 Campbell MJ and Machin D (1999) *Medical Statistics: a common-sense approach* (3e). Wiley, Chichester.
7 Bowers D (2002) *Statistics From Scratch: an introduction for health care professionals* (2e). Wiley, Chichester.
8 Altman DG, Machin D, Bryant TN and Gardner MJ (eds) (2000) *Statistics With Confidence* (2e). BMJ Books, London.
9 Kinnear PR and Gray CD (2004) *SPSS 12 Made Simple* (1e). Psychology Press, East Sussex.

Chapter 19

Significance tests and others

Introduction

Choosing an appropriate significance test for statistical analysis of data is of utmost importance. The selection of an appropriate statistical test depends on:

- sample size
- distribution of data and
- type of data (paired/unpaired or nominal/ordinal/numerical).

Statistical significance tests are of two types – parametric and non-parametric tests.

Parametric tests

These are used with the data assumed to have a Normal distribution, which could be characterised by a few parameters like the *mean* and *standard deviation*. Parametric tests thus use the *distributional assumption* and can describe the theoretical distribution by parameters like *mean* and *standard deviation*. Examples are:

- *The t-test* – also known as *Student's t-test* for the pseudonym 'Student' used by the originator of the *t*-test, WS Gosset (1876–1937), who showed that the mean of a sample from a Normal distribution with unknown variance has a distribution similar to, but not quite the same as, a Normal distribution and he called it *t* distribution (*see* Appendices 2 and 4).
- *The z-test* – used to calculate the *z*-score to determine the p-value, as described earlier.
- *Pearson's coefficient of linear correlation (r).*

If the sample size is large with an assumed Normal distribution in the population (however, lack of normality is of less concern if the sample size is large) and the data are numerical, then calculation of the *mean, SD, SEM, confidence interval* and *p-value*, from the table of Normal distribution, are all that we need to assess the statistical significance of the study results. However, with a small sample (usually < 30), we have to use *t* distribution rather than Normal distribution (i.e. using the *t* score to get the p-value from the table of *t* distribution, rather than using the *z*-score to get the p-value from the table of Normal distribution) to get a reliable result. As, with a large sample, *t*-score and *z*-score give similar p-values (actually these two scores are the same if the sample size is ∞), there is no justification for using Normal distribution for a large sample. It is rather simpler to use the same *t* distribution for both small and large samples.

Non-parametric tests

These are used for the data which do not have a Normal distribution and cannot be characterised by a few parameters, which is somewhat of a misnomer. As these tests do not use any distributional assumption and cannot be described by parameters like mean and standard deviation, they are known as *distribution-free* or *non-parametric* methods. These tests are based on *analysis of rank or order* of data and are known as *rank score tests*. Examples are:

- *Sign test.*
- *Wilcoxon test* (conventionally for paired data).
- *Mann–Whitney U-test* (conventionally for unpaired data).
- *Spearman's rank correlation (r_s).*
- *Chi-squared (χ^2) test* – this test can be carried out only on the actual number of occurrences, not on percentages, proportions, means of observations or other derived statistics (*see* Appendices 3 and 5).
- *McNemar's test* – a special form of χ^2-test used in the analysis of paired proportions (e.g. before and after test).

It can be argued that since non-parametric tests are distribution-free, they should be used always. However, the overwhelming arguments against the routine use of non-parametric tests are that they are *not flexible enough* and *less powerful* when used with data with a normal distribution.

Similar to parametric methods, non-parametric methods use various tables of distribution like F distribution, χ^2 distribution, etc.

Choice of significance test

The choice of a suitable statistical significance test for hypothesis testing depends on a variety of factors, mainly the study hypothesis and the type of data (independent/paired, nominal/ordinal/numerical).

While each case should be considered on its own merits, a rough guide in choosing a test is as follows.

Comparing groups – continuous data

- **For one group of observations** – to compare with a set standard or specific hypothesised mean.
  - parametric test: *one-sample t-test*
  - equivalent non-parametric tests: *Sign test* or *Wilcoxon signed rank sum test.*
- **For two groups of paired observations** – to compare two sets of observations on a single sample.
  - parametric test: *paired t-test*
  - equivalent non-parametric tests: *Sign test* or *Wilcoxon matched pairs signed rank sum test.*
- **For two independent groups of observations** – to compare two independent samples drawn from the same population. To determine whether two samples are drawn from the same population, we may have to perform the F test or variance ratio test.

- parametric test: *two-samples t-test*
- equivalent non-parametric test: *Mann–Whitney U-test*.
- **For skewed data** – taking logarithms of data with skewed distribution often transforms into near-normal distribution.
  - parametric test: *paired t-test of the logs of data*
  - equivalent non-parametric test: *Wilcoxon matched pairs signed rank sum test on the raw data*.
- **For three or more independent groups of observations:**
  - parametric test: *one-way analysis of variance (ANOVA) (e.g. F test)*
  - equivalent non-parametric test: *Kruskal–Wallis test*.
- **Strength of association between two continuous variables:**
  - parametric test: *Pearson's coefficient of linear correlation (r)*
  - equivalent non-parametric test: *Spearman's rank correlation (r$_s$)*.
- **Numerical relationship between two or more continuous variables:**
  - *regression* or *multiple regression by least squares method*.
- **Relation between several variables:**
  - *two way or multiple analysis of variance (MANOVA)*.

Comparing groups – categorical data

Analysis of categorical data can be done either by *frequency table approach* or *comparison of proportions*. The frequency table approach is commonly used and it is suitable for larger tables containing multiple categories as well. However, the comparison of proportions is preferable as it readily yields p-values and confidence intervals.

Frequency tables are also known as *contingency tables* or *r* (row) × *c* (column) tables. The combinations of row and column categories are known as *cells*. The expected value in a cell is calculated with the following formula: expected value *(E)* = total of the row in which the cell lies multiplied by total of the column in which the cell lies and then dividing the result by the sample size *(n)*. So:

$$E = (\text{row total} \times \text{column total})/n$$

This is applicable to contingency tables of any size. The analysis of frequency tables is largely based on hypothesis testing.

- For two paired proportions: *McNemar's test*.
- For two or more independent proportions: *Chi-squared (χ^2) test*.
- For ordered categories: *Chi-squared (χ^2) test for trend* or *Mann–Whitney U-test*.
- For small samples with very small expected frequencies (< 80% of cells have expected value of at least 5): *Fisher's exact test*.[1–3]

Sample size estimation

Sample size estimation is a crucial point in designing a trial for statistical power of the study. If the sample size is too small it will not be able to answer the question posed and the patients may be put at risk with no benefit but a waste of time and money. On the other hand too large a sample will cause a waste of resources.

Estimation of required sample size, to get a statistically significant and reliable result, depends on the following factors:

- type of data and study design
- significance level (α)
- expected power of the study $(1 - \beta)$
- variance (SD^2) of the data (σ^2)
- effect size or difference of interest (d), the minimum difference that would be clinically significant.

Sample size estimation can be done by complicated formulae (*see* Campbell and Machin 1999 and Appendix 7)[2] or by a much simpler graphic method using a nomogram (*see* Altman and Gore 1982 and Appendix 6).[1,4]

In the graphic method, the left-hand column of the nomogram represents a scale of *standardised difference* (the ratio of the difference of interest (d) to the standard deviation (s), i.e. $d/s = z$-score). The right-hand column of the nomogram is a scale for *expected power of the study $(1 - \beta)$* and the middle column represents necessary *sample size (N) at two levels of significance* $(\alpha = 0.05$ or $0.01)$. When we connect the appropriate points on the two scales (left and right) by a straight line, then this line cuts the middle column of the nomogram at two points which represent necessary sample size at two different significance levels.[1,4]

Survival analysis

Survival analysis deals with a particular type of data, which arises when our interest is focused on the time taken for some event to occur. Because this type of study was originally concerned with survival (at the end of a specific follow-up period after a particular surgical procedure or diagnosis of a particular disease), it is named as *survival study* and the data arising from this type of study are called *survival data*. Apart from mortality, similar data can arise from a variety of situations, such as time taken to develop a particular symptom or disease, time taken to maximum exercise tolerance, time for a leg fracture to heal, time that a transdermal patch can be left in place, etc. Conventionally we stick to the same terminology of 'survival data' to describe these data as well.

As there is usually a fixed follow-up period, we cannot wait until the final events have happened to all the subjects and some patients may even be lost to follow-up within that fixed period. Thus the only information we have about some patients is that they were still alive at the last follow-up and this leads to *censored observations*.

If there is no censored observation, we may not necessarily have to use survival analysis; we can use a rank score test like the Mann–Whitney U-test. However, in survival analysis we analyse the censored data using a *Kaplan–Meier survival curve* (a plot of cumulative survival probability against time).

The probability of surviving a given length of time can be calculated by considering time in many small intervals. The probability of a patient surviving two days after a procedure can be considered to be the probability of surviving the first day (P_1), multiplied by the probability of surviving the second day (P_2) given that the patient survived the first day. This second probability is called *conditional probability*. Similarly, if P_{100} is the probability of surviving the hundredth day,

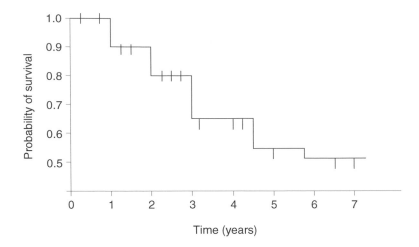

Figure 19.1 Example Kaplan–Meier survival curve.

conditional on having already survived the first 99 days, then the overall 100 days survival probability = $P_1 \times P_2 \dots \dots P_{99} \times P_{100}$.

The survival curve is drawn as a *step function*: the proportion surviving remains unchanged between events, i.e. although there are some intermediate censored observations, they are calculated only at the end of each time interval as if all those observations took place at the very end of that interval period. It is incorrect to join the calculated points by sloping lines instead of stepwise fashion. The time of censored observations is sometimes indicated by ticks or vertical lines on the survival curve. For example, the probability of survival of a group of patients with colorectal cancer, followed up over a period of seven years, is shown in the *Kaplan–Meier survival curve* in Figure 19.1.

Comparison between two survival curves from two groups is usually done by a *log rank test*, which is a non-parametric method of hypothesis testing. The principle of the log rank test is to divide the survival timescale into intervals according to the distinct observed survival times and the censored survival times are ignored. Unlike many other life tables, here the time intervals are not of equal length.

We can use *hazard ratio (HR)* to measure relative survival in two groups, provided the calculation is based on the complete period studied.

We can use the log rank test for comparing the survival experience of two or more groups. However, it cannot be used to explore the effects of several variables on survival. To study the effects of several variables on survival, we need a method similar to multiple regression analysis, known as *proportional hazards regression analysis*. This is an extension of the log rank test and also known as *Cox regression*, after the name of Cox, who introduced this method first in 1972.[1,5,6]

References

1   Altman DG (1991) *Practical Statistics for Medical Research*. Chapman and Hall/CRC, London.
2   Campbell MJ and Machin D (1999) *Medical Statistics: a common-sense approach* (3e). Wiley, Chichester.
3   Armitage P and Berry G (1994) *Statistical Methods in Medical Research* (3e). Blackwell Science, Oxford.
4   Altman DG and Gore SM (eds) (1982) *Statistics in Practice*. BMA, London.
5   Swinscow TDV and Campbell MJ (2002) *Statistics at Square One* (10e). BMJ Books, London.
6   Bowers D (2002) *Statistics From Scratch: an introduction for health care professionals* (2e). Wiley, Chichester.

Chapter 20

Diagnostic statistics

Diagnostic statistics play a significant role in various diagnostic testing or screening tests and in our day-to-day practice of clinical medicine. The following are a few commonly used terms in diagnostic statistics.

Gold standard test – refers to a *valid* diagnostic tool, which consistently gives the correct diagnosis, i.e. is *reliable* and *accurate*. In practice, gold standards are rarely 100% accurate, but they are simply the *best* method of diagnosis according to current dogma. Gold standard tests are often *invasive* or *expensive*, but can be used in studies to assess the performance (i.e. sensitivity and specificity) of simpler and/or cheaper methods.

Incidence – of a disease is a measure of the number of *new cases* of the disease occurring during a specified period of time and is expressed with reference to the *person-time at risk* (e.g. 5 per 1000 persons per year).

Prevalence – of a disease is a measure of the total number of *existing cases* of the disease at a particular point in time (point prevalence) or a specified time period (period prevalence), divided by the total population or by the total population at the midpoint of the specified interval. It is expressed per 100, 1000 or 100 000 depending on the degree of prevalence. In the context of diagnostic testing, prevalence is often used as an estimate of the *pre-test probability* of disease.

Probability – is the estimation of the likely prevalence of a condition or outcome of an intervention based on previous experience or an educated guess. Probability is assessed by one of three approaches: the *frequency* approach, *model-based* approach and *subjective* approach.

Contingency tables (2 × 2) – are used to summarise the association between two categorical variables or binary variables. *Two columns* represent the different levels of one variable and the *two rows* represent the different levels of another variable. This is a very important tool used to summarise data in an *observational study*, *clinical trial* and *diagnostic testing*.

For example, Table 20.1 shows a contingency table in the context of *diagnostic testing*.

Table 20.1 Contingency table for diagnostic testing

| | | Diseased | | |
		Yes	*No*	*Total*
	Positive	a	b	a + b
Test result	Negative	c	d	c + d
	Total	a + c	b + d	a + b + c + d

Sensitivity – measures how good a test is in detecting those individuals who are truly diseased, i.e. detection of the *true positives* or *true positive rate (TPR)*. ∴ Sensitivity = all testing positive and diseased/all diseased = $a/(a + c)$. The complement of sensitivity, i.e. (1 – sensitivity), is the *false negative rate (FNR)* = $1 - a/(a + c) = c/(a + c)$.

Specificity – measures how good a test is in detecting those individuals who are not diseased, i.e. detection of the *true negatives* or *true negative rate (TNR)*. ∴ Specificity = all testing negative and non-diseased/all non-diseased = $d/(b + d)$. The complement of specificity, i.e. (1 – specificity), is the *false positive rate (FPR)* = $1 - d/(b + d) = b/(b + d)$.

Both sensitivity and specificity are not usually affected by the change in prevalence of the disease in question.

Accuracy – indicates what proportion of all tests gives correct result; i.e. *true positives and true negatives* as a proportion of all tests = $(a + d)/(a + b + c + d)$.

Positive predictive value (PPV) – the PPV of a test is the probability of actually having a condition given that the test result is positive. ∴ *PPV* = all testing positive and diseased/all testing positive = $a/(a + b)$.

Negative predictive value (NPV) – the NPV of a test is the probability of not having the condition given that the test result is negative. ∴ *NPV* = all testing negative and non-diseased/all testing negative = $d/(c + d)$.

Predictive values measure how useful a test is in practice and they are affected by changes in disease prevalence. A higher prevalence results in an increased PPV and a lower prevalence results in a decreased PPV. The opposite is true for the NPV.

Likelihood ratio (LR) – the LR expresses the likelihood of finding the test result in patients with the condition relative to the likelihood of the same test result in patients without the condition.

∴ *(+) LR* = likelihood of +ve test result among diseased/likelihood of +ve test result among non-diseased = $\{a/(a + c)\}/\{b/(b + d)\}$ = *TPR/FPR*. A (+) LR > 1 is a good test for positive results, i.e. a positive result is more likely to be a true positive than a false positive.

∴ *(–) LR* – likelihood of –ve test result among diseased/likelihood of –ve test result among non-diseased = $\{c/(a + c)\}/\{d/(b + d)\}$ = *FNR/TNR*. A (–) LR < 1 is a good test for negative results, i.e. a negative result is more likely to be a true negative than a false negative.

Relative (receiver) operating characteristics (ROC) – when a diagnostic test produces a continuous measurement, then a convenient diagnostic cut-off must be selected to calculate the sensitivity and specificity of the test. For every possible cut-off value there will be a corresponding sensitivity and specificity. We can display these calculations by graphing the *sensitivity* (true positives) on the y-axis (vertical) and the false positive rate *(1 – specificity)* on the x-axis (horizontal) for all possible cut-off values of the diagnostic test. The resulting curve is known as the *relative (receiver) operating characteristic curve* or *ROC curve*.

The ROC curve demonstrates the trade-off between sensitivity and specificity as the threshold for test positivity is changed. A perfect diagnostic test would be

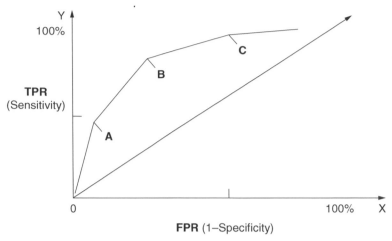

Figure 20.1 Example ROC curve. **A**: high threshold for +ve; **C**: low threshold for +ve; **B** is a reasonable compromise between sensitivity and specificity.

one with no false-positive or false-negative results and would be represented by a line that starts at the origin and goes up the y-axis to a sensitivity of 1, and then across to a false positive rate of 0. A test with a $TPR = FPR$ would produce a ROC curve on the diagonal line $y = x$. Any reasonable diagnostic test should have a $TPR > FPR$ and would display a ROC curve in the upper left triangle of the graph (for example, *see* Figure 20.1).

Table 20.2 shows a contingency table in the context of *clinical trials* and *observational studies*.

Table 20.2 Contingency table for clinical trials and observational studies

| | | *Exposure/intervention* | | |
		Yes	*No*	*Total*
Study	Positive	a	b	a + b
outcome	Negative	c	d	c + d
	Total	a + c	b + d	a + b + c + d

Risk (R) and risk ratio or relative risk (RR) – means the probability of occurrence of an event within some given time period; these are used in *prospective studies*. *Risk (R)* = number of events/number of people at risk = $(a + b)/(a + b + c + d)$. *Relative risk (RR)* = risk in exposed group/risk in control group = $\{a/(a + c)\}/\{b/b + d)\}$.

Hazard ratio (HR) – is the measure of *relative risk* used in *survival* studies. It is calculated as: $HR = (O_1/E_1)/(O_2/E_2)$ where O_1 and O_2 are the *observed* number of subjects with the event in groups 1 and 2 respectively; and E_1 and E_2 are the *expected* number of subjects with the event in groups 1 and 2 respectively. A HR of 1 means the hazard or risk of the event is the same in the two groups being compared. A HR less than 1 suggests group 1 is less likely to experience the event than group 2 and the opposite is true if the HR is greater than 1.

Odds and odds ratio (OR) – these terms are used in *case control (retrospective) studies* instead of risk and relative risk respectively.

- *Odds* = ratio of number of times an event occurs (P) to number of times it does not occur (1– P) = $P/(1 - P)$.
- *Odds ratio (OR)* = odds in the exposed/odds in the non-exposed = $a/c : b/d = ad/bc$.

For rare diseases the OR and RR will be very similar. For a common event, e.g. a newborn baby being a boy or a girl, the probability or risk is roughly 0.5 or 50%, but the odds is 1 (50:50).

An OR = 1 means that there is no difference between two groups whereas an OR < 1 is significant in favour of treatment or intervention.

Absolute risk difference or reduction (ARD or ARR) – in comparative studies ARR expresses the benefit of one treatment or intervention compared with the other. It is also known as *attributable risk*. If the risk in the study group is R_1 and the risk in the control group is R_2 then: $ARR = R_2 - R_1 = b/(b + d) - a/(a + c)$.

Relative risk reduction (RRR) – RRR is interpreted as the proportion of the initial or baseline risk, which was eliminated by the given treatment or intervention, or by avoidance of exposure or a risk factor. So: $RRR = (1 - RR) \times 100\%$.

Number needed to treat (NNT) – this is a measure of the impact of a treatment or intervention. It states how many patients need to be treated with the treatment in question, in order to prevent an event which would otherwise occur. So: $NNT = 1/(R_2 - R_1) = 1/ARR$.[1-3]

References

1   Altman DG (1991) *Practical Statistics for Medical Research*. Chapman and Hall/CRC, London.
2   Swinscow TDV and Campbell MJ (2002) *Statistics at Square One* (10e). BMJ Books, London.
3   Pereira-Maxwell F (1998) *A–Z of Medical Statistics: a companion for critical appraisal*. Arnold, London.

Appendices

Appendices 1, 2 and 3 include tables for p-value estimation for normal distribution, t distribution and χ^2 distribution respectively. For detailed and extensive tables the reader is referred to any standard textbook on statistics.

P-value (two-sided) table for normal distribution (z → p)

Example – the two-sided p-value corresponding to $z = 2.00$ is 0.045, which is < 0.050 and statistically significant.

z-score	p-value
0.00	**1.00**
0.10	0.92
0.20	0.84
0.30	0.76
0.40	0.69
0.50	0.62
0.60	0.55
0.674	**0.500**
0.70	0.48
0.80	0.42
0.90	0.37
1.00	*0.31*
1.10	0.27
1.20	0.23
1.30	0.19
1.40	0.16
1.50	0.13
1.60	0.11
1.645	**0.100**
1.70	0.089
1.80	0.072
1.90	0.057
1.960	**0.050**
2.00	*0.045*
2.10	0.036
2.20	0.028
2.30	0.021
2.40	0.016
2.50	0.012
2.576	**0.010**
3.00	*0.0027*
3.291	0.0010
3.891	0.00010
4.00	*0.00006*

The *t* distribution for two-tailed p-value estimation (*t* → p)

To be significant at a particular level of significance, the sample *t*-value must be greater than the corresponding tabulated value (*t-score*) below (as the higher the *t*-score, the lower the p-value).

Example – the two-tailed (sided) p-value corresponding to an observed test statistic *t* = 2.810 (which is > 2.787) for 25 degrees of freedom is < 0.01 (0.001 < p < 0.01).

Degree of freedom	0.10	0.05	p-value 0.02	0.01	0.001
1	6.314	12.706	31.821	63.657	636.619
2	2.920	4.303	6.965	9.925	31.598
3	2.353	3.182	4.541	5.841	12.941
4	2.132	2.776	3.747	4.604	8.610
5	2.015	2.571	3.365	4.032	6.859
6	1.943	2.447	3.143	3.707	5.959
7	1.895	2.365	2.998	3.499	5.405
8	1.860	2.306	2.896	3.355	5.041
9	1.833	2.262	2.821	3.250	4.781
10	1.812	2.228	2.764	3.169	4.587
11	1.796	2.201	2.718	3.106	4.437
12	1.782	2.179	2.681	3.055	4.318
13	1.771	2.160	2.650	3.012	4.221
14	1.761	2.145	2.624	2.977	4.140
15	1.753	2.131	2.602	2.947	4.073
16	1.746	2.120	2.583	2.921	4.015
17	1.740	2.110	2.567	2.898	3.965
18	1.734	2.101	2.552	2.878	3.922
19	1.729	2.093	2.539	2.861	3.883
20	1.725	2.086	2.528	2.845	3.850
21	1.721	2.080	2.518	2.831	3.819
22	1.717	2.074	2.508	2.819	3.792
23	1.714	2.069	2.500	2.807	3.767
24	1.711	2.064	2.492	2.797	3.745
25	1.708	2.060	2.485	2.787	3.725
26	1.706	2.056	2.479	2.779	3.707
27	1.703	2.052	2.473	2.771	3.690
28	1.701	2.048	2.467	2.763	3.674
29	1.699	2.045	2.462	2.756	3.659
30	1.697	2.042	2.457	2.750	3.646

40	1.684	2.021	2.432	2.704	3.551
50	*1.676*	*2.009*	*2.403*	*2.678*	*3.496*
60	1.671	2.000	2.390	2.660	3.460
70	1.667	1.994	2.381	2.648	3.435
80	1.664	1.990	2.374	2.639	3.416
90	1.662	1.987	2.368	2.632	3.402
100	*1.660*	*1.984*	*2.364*	*2.626*	*3.390*
∞	1.645	1.960	2.326	2.576	3.291

Chi-squared (χ^2) distribution for two-tailed p-value estimation ($\chi^2 \rightarrow$ p)

The p-value will be less than the tabulated value, if the value of the test statistic X^2 is greater than the corresponding tabulated value of χ^2 (as the higher the value of χ^2, the lower the p-value).

Example – the two-tailed p-value corresponding to an observed test statistic $X^2 = 31.450$ on 20 degrees of freedom is < 0.05 ($0.02 < p < 0.05$).

			p-value		
Degree of freedom	*0.10*	*0.05*	*0.02*	*0.01*	*0.001*
1	2.706	3.841	5.412	6.635	10.827
2	4.605	5.991	7.824	9.210	13.815
3	6.251	7.815	9.837	11.345	16.268
4	7.779	9.488	11.668	13.277	18.465
5	*9.236*	*11.070*	*13.388*	*15.086*	*20.517*
6	10.645	12.592	15.033	16.812	22.457
7	12.017	14.067	16.622	18.475	24.322
8	13.362	15.507	18.168	20.090	26.125
9	14.684	16.919	19.679	21.666	27.877
10	*15.987*	*18.307*	*21.161*	*23.209*	*29.588*
11	17.275	19.675	22.618	24.725	31.264
12	18.549	21.026	24.054	26.217	32.909
13	19.812	22.362	25.472	27.688	34.528
14	21.064	23.685	26.873	29.141	36.123
15	*22.307*	*24.996*	*28.259*	*30.578*	*37.697*
16	23.542	26.296	29.633	32.000	39.252
17	24.769	27.587	30.995	33.409	40.790
18	25.989	28.869	32.346	34.805	42.312
19	27.204	30.144	33.687	36.191	43.820
20	*28.412*	*31.410*	*35.020*	*37.566*	*45.315*
21	29.615	32.671	36.343	38.932	46.797
22	30.813	33.924	37.659	40.289	48.268
23	32.007	35.172	38.968	41.638	49.728
24	33.196	36.415	40.270	42.980	51.179
25	*34.382*	*37.652*	*41.566*	*44.314*	*52.620*
26	35.563	38.885	42.856	45.642	54.052
27	36.741	40.113	44.140	46.963	55.476
28	37.916	41.337	45.419	48.278	56.893
29	39.087	42.557	46.693	49.588	58.302
30	*40.256*	*43.773*	*47.962*	*50.892*	*59.703*

Student's *t*-test

Student's *t*-test is a very commonly used parametric test. Being a parametric test it uses the distributional assumption that the data (means, proportions or differences between means or proportions) are normally distributed. As discussed under parametric tests in Chapter 19, the *t*-test is more useful for a small sample size, but for simplistic reasons it is used for both small and large samples.

The *t*-test also uses a particular parameter called *degrees of freedom (df)* to get more accurate results. In general the degrees of freedom is calculated as sample size minus the number of estimated parameters.

The test statistic *t* is calculated using the same formula used with normal distribution as follows:

> test statistic *t* = the ratio of the *quantity of interest* to its *standard error* =
> [sample mean (*x*) − hypothesised mean (*k*)]/standard error of mean (*SE*)

So, $t = (x − k)/(SD/\sqrt{n})$ [as standard error of mean *(SE)* = standard deviation of mean *(SD)* divided by the square root of sample size *(n)*]. The only difference is that we have to find the result in a table of *t* distribution, using appropriate degrees of freedom, rather than the table of normal distribution.

There are three types of *t*-test as follows:

1   *One-sample t-test* – used to compare the sample mean *(x)* with specific hypothesised mean *(k)* (e.g. postulated population mean). The value of the test statistic *t* is calculated with the formula: $t = (x − k)/(SD/\sqrt{n})$ and the confidence interval is calculated as usual with the formula: 95% CI = mean ± *t* value as per degree of freedom × standard error of mean = $x ± t_{n−1} × (SE)$.
    Example – the recommended daily intake of calcium in young adults is 1 gram (1000 mg). In a study of ten young adults we found that their daily calcium intake during summer and winter seasons was as shown in Table A4.1.
    Now, if we want to study the difference of mean daily calcium intake in the summer season with the daily recommended level, by using a *one-sample t-test*, then:

$$t = (850 − 1000)/(156.33/\sqrt{10}) = − (150/49.336) = −3.040.$$

Now we can find the *p-value* from the table of *t* distribution with a degree of freedom of (10 − 1) = 9 and we can ignore the sign of *t* for a two-sided test. The result shows $0.01 < p < 0.02$, which is statistically significant and does not support the null hypothesis that there is no difference between the observed level and the recommended level of daily calcium intake; it rather suggests that the dietary intake of these young adults was significantly less than the recommended level. The 95% CI = 850 ± 2.262 × 49.336 = 850 ± 112 = *738 to 962* (as the value of *t* = 2.262 at *9* degrees of freedom for *p* = 0.05 and

Table A4.1 Daily calcium intake

Subject	Daily calcium intake (mg)		
	Summer season	*Winter season*	*Difference*
1	600	700	100
2	650	725	75
3	700	775	75
4	750	800	50
5	800	850	50
6	850	875	25
7	900	950	50
8	950	1000	50
9	1050	1125	75
10	1250	1300	50
Mean	850	910	60
SD	*156.33*	*188.41*	*21.08*

SE = 49.336), which means that there is 95% probability of the true population mean to lie within this range.

2 *Paired t-test* – used to study the difference between means of paired samples, where the differences have a presumed normal distribution. The test is derived from the one-sample *t*-test, where we compare the mean of observed differences (d) with a hypothesised value of zero difference (0), as the null hypothesis is that there is no difference between the paired observations. So:

$$t = (d - 0)/SE(d) = d/SE(d) \text{ and } 95\% \text{ CI} = d \pm t_{n-1} \times SE(d)$$
$$[SE(d) = \text{the standard error of the mean difference (d)}]$$

Example – from the above example if we want to compare the daily calcium intake in summer and winter seasons, then we have to use a *paired t-test* and so, $t = 60/(21.08/\sqrt{10}) = 60/6.666 = 9.000$. Now, from the table of *t* distribution for a degree of freedom of 9, we can get the *p-value* of $p < 0.001$, which is highly significant and does not support the null hypothesis; rather it suggests that the difference between calcium intake in summer and winter seasons in this paired sample is significant. The 95% confidence interval is: $60 \pm 2.262 \times 6.666 = 60 \pm 15 = 45 \text{ to } 75$, which means that there is 95% probability of the true population mean difference to lie within this range.

3 *Two samples t-test* – is used to study the difference between the means of two independent samples, where the means are different but the standard deviations of the samples are the same. (If the standard deviations are markedly different then one of the assumptions of the *t*-test, that the two samples come from populations with the same standard deviation, is unlikely to hold and we have to use another appropriate test [e.g. Welsh's test] rather than the *t*-test.)

The value of the test statistic *t* is calculated with the following formula:

$$t = (x_1 - x_2)/SE(x_1 - x_2)$$

where x_1 and x_2 are the means of two samples and $SE(x_1 - x_2)$ is the standard error of mean.

The calculation of confidence interval in this test needs a parameter called *pooled variance* (s_p^2), which is derived from a complicated equation:

- pooled variance = (s_p^2) = $\{(n_1 - 1)s_1^2 + (n_2 - 1)s_2^2\}/(n_1 + n_2 - 2)$
- standard error of mean = SE $(x_1 - x_2)$ = $\sqrt{\{(s_p^2 / n_1) + (s_p^2 / n_2)\}}$
- confidence interval (CI) = $(x_1 - x_2) \pm t_{(n1 + n2 - 2)}$ SE $(x_1 - x_2)$.

where x_1 and x_2 are the means of two samples, n_1 and n_2 are respective sample sizes, s_1 and s_2 are respective standard deviations and $(n_1 + n_2 - 2)$ is the degree of freedom.

Example – we can use the above example if we consider that those two samples were not paired; rather, they were two independent samples taken at the same time. *(In this case, unlike the above example, the sample sizes are usually unequal and the last column in the above example showing differences between paired observations does not exist.)*

Now, by using the *two-samples t-test*, we can calculate the value of *t* as follows:

- (s_p^2) = $\{(10 - 1) \times (156.33)^2 + (10 - 1) \times (188.41)^2\}/(10 + 10 - 2)$ = $\{9 (24444.444 + 35500)\}/18$ = 29972.222 and
- SE $(x_1 - x_2)$ = $\sqrt{\{(29972.222/10) + (29972.222/10)\}}$ = 77.423 and so
- t = $(x_1 - x_2)/$SE $(x_1 - x_2)$ = $(850 - 910)/77.423$ = $- 0.775$.

The p-value from the table of *t*-distribution for 18 degrees of freedom is: *p* > *0.10*, which is not significant and supports the null hypothesis that there is no difference in calcium intake between the two groups.

The *95% CI = 60 ± 2.101 × 77.423* (as the value of *t* = 2.101 at *18* degrees of freedom for a *p = 0.05*) = *−102.665 to +222.665 or (−) 103 to (+) 223*, which is very wide and includes the value of no difference *(0)* and so is not significant.

In this example, both the p-value and confidence interval are insignificant, suggesting that there is no significant difference in calcium intake between these two independent groups.

Appendix 5

Chi-squared (χ^2) test

If a variable X has a standard Normal distribution, then X^2 has a distribution which is known as Chi-squared (χ^2) distribution. Conventionally, for the sample statistic we use the Latin (X^2) and for the test and distribution we use the Greek (χ^2). Obviously, X^2 can only have positive values and the distribution is highly skewed. Like t distribution, Chi-squared distribution also uses the parameter *degree of freedom (df)*. In the simplest case, the χ^2 distribution with one degree of freedom is simply the square of a standard Normal distribution, so the 5% cut-off point for X^2 is the square of the 5% cut-off point for the Normal distribution, i.e. 1.96^2 or 3.84.

As X^2 can have only positive values, it represents only the upper tail of the χ^2 distribution, which corresponds to both tails of the standard Normal distribution. When the Chi-squared test is used for analysis of a frequency table, the number of degrees of freedom is the product of $(r - 1)(c - 1)$, where r and c represent the number of rows and columns respectively.

The conventional criterion for validity of a χ^2 test is attributed to the great statistician WG Cochran. The *rule* is: the χ^2 test is valid if at least 80% of the expected frequencies exceed 5 and all the expected frequencies exceed 1. The expected frequency (E) in any particular cell of a frequency table is calculated with the formula: $E = (row\ total \times column\ total)/n$.

Chi-squared test is used to analyse categorical data arising from single, two or more independent samples for detecting any relationship between different categories of a single sample or between variables from different samples. In case of a *single sample*, the test compares the observed values (O) with a hypothesised or expected value (E) and the test is called a *Chi-squared goodness-of-fit test*.

Steps in performing a Chi-squared test

Step 1: Find the observed value in each category *(O)*.
Step 2: Determine the expected value in each category *(E)*.
Step 3: Calculate *(O − E)* value for each category.
Step 4: Square each of the above values $[(O - E)^2]$.
Step 5: Standardise the above value by dividing it with E for that category $[(O - E)^2/E]$.
Step 6: Sum all the values from the step above to get the value of the test statistic (X^2). So: $X^2 = \Sigma\,[(O - E)^2/E]$.

Now, we have to use this (X^2) value to get the *p-value* from the table of (χ^2) distribution, for an appropriate degree of freedom (*see* Appendix 3). The *p-value*, thus calculated, will determine whether the study (null) hypothesis is true or false.